Nutrition in the
20th Century

Myron Winick, Editor

Institute of Human Nutrition
Columbia University College of Physicians and Surgeons

Volume 1:   Nutrition and Development
Volume 2:   Nutrition and Fetal Development
Volume 3:   Childhood Obesity
Volume 4:   Nutrition and Aging
Volume 5:   Nutritional Disorders of American Women
Volume 6:   Nutrition and Cancer
Volume 7:   Hunger Disease: Studies by the Jewish
            Physicians in the Warsaw Ghetto
Volume 8:   Nutritional Management of Genetic Disorders
Volume 9:   Nutrition and Gastroenterology
Volume 10: Nutrition and the Killer Diseases
Volume 11: Adolescent Nutrition
Volume 12: Nutrition and Drugs
Volume 13: Nutrition in the 20th Century

NUTRITION IN THE 20TH CENTURY

Edited by

MYRON WINICK
Institute of Human Nutrition
Columbia University College of
Physicians and Surgeons

A WILEY-INTERSCIENCE PUBLICATION
JOHN WILEY & SONS
New York · Chichester · Brisbane · Toronto · Singapore

Library of Congress Cataloging in Publication Data
Main entry under title:

Nutrition in the 20th century.

  (Current concepts in nutrition, ISSN 0090-0443 ; v. 13)
  "A Wiley-Interscience publication."
  Includes index.
  1. Nutrition. I. Winick, Myron. II. Series. [DNLM:
1. Nutrition. W1 CU788AS v.13 / QU 145 N97534]
QP141.N794 1984   613.2   84-13044
ISBN 0-471-81165-3

Printed in the United States of America

10 9 8 7 6 5 4 3 2 1

Preface

In many ways the 20th Century might be called the century of science. We have come from the horse and wagon to men on the moon, from steam generated power to nuclear power, from telegraph to television. In the biological sciences the discoveries leading up to genetic engineering have set us on the brink of a whole new era. Although perhaps less dramatic, the history of nutrition in the 20th Century has been extremely exciting. In the early part of the century the discovery of vitamins, their action, and their role in maintaining health dominated the field. In the later part of the century the role of diet in preventing chronic disease has assumed prominence. This volume both reviews the history of nutrition in the 20th Century and discusses the most recent work in the context of earlier discoveries. It brings us up to date on research dealing with vitamins and minerals and covers what is currently known about nutrition in both prenatal and postnatal development. Finally, one of the most serious diseases related directly to nutrition, obesity, is discussed in the light of the most recent results.

There are still 15 years left in the 20th Century and 15 years can be a long time in the life of a science. The final portion of this volume deals with areas of nutrition still in their infancy but destined, in my opinion, to be among the most exciting areas in the coming decade and a half. The mysteries involved in nutrient control of behavior are rapidly being unraveled. The newest type of nutrition, which bypasses the gastrointestinal tract, total parenteral nutrition, is discussed as a vehicle for studying single nutrient action under a variety of conditions. By the end of this century more than 20% of our population will be 65 or over. We have only recently focused on this population from the standpoint of nutrition. Already a great deal of new information is available. Perhaps our greatest challenge in the next 15 years is to eliminate cancer as a major disease. Whether this is accomplished or not, the role of nutrition in the cause of various cancers has become well recognized and will assume more importance as we gather more information. Thus, the chapters on the elderly and on nutrition and cancer attempt to bridge the gap between the present and the future and outline the direction research is heading in these two important areas. This book, unlike its predecessors, is not organized around a single subject area. Instead it highlights several areas—areas that have been important, remain important, and almost certainly will continue to be important for the rest of this century and beyond.

Myron Winick, M.D.

New York, New York
August, 1984

Contents

1. The First Fifty Years   1
    Elsie M. Widdowson, F.R.S., D.Sc.

2. Ascorbic Acid as it Relates to the Metabolism of Drugs
    and Environmental Agents   21
    V. G. Zannoni, R. L. Susick, and R. C. Smart

3. Trace Metals in Human Nutrition   37
    Harold H. Sandstead, M.D.

4. Nutrition During Pregnancy: Myths and Realities   47
    P. Rosso, M.D.

5. Nutrition and Brain Development   71
    Myron Winick, M.D.

6. Thermogenesis in Human Obesity   87
    F. Xavier Pi-Sunyer, M.D.

7. Effects of Foods and Nutrients on Brain
    Neurotransmitters   103
    Richard J. Wurtman, M.D.

8. The Assessment of the Functional Consequences of
    Malnutrition   113
    David McR. Russell, MBBS, FRACP, and Khursheed N.
    Jeejeebhoy, MBBS, Ph.D., FRCP(C)

9. Nutrition and Aging   137
    S. Jaime Rozovski, Ph.D.

10. Nutrition, Diet and Cancer—An Evaluation   171
Ernst L. Wynder, M.D.

Index   195

1

The First Fifty Years

ELSIE M. WIDDOWSON, F.R.S., D.Sc.

Department of Medicine, Addenbrooke's Hospital, Cambridge, England

ENERGY METABOLISM

My story must begin with Atwater. Atwater tends to be forgotten nowadays, but he was responsible for introducing the science of nutrition into the United States. The study of energy metabolism had its origins in France at the end of the 18th Century, but by the middle of the 19th Century the scene had shifted to Germany, and three important names are Rubner, Voit, and Pettenkoffer. Rubner analyzed foods for water, nitrogen, and fat and assumed the remainder to be carbohydrate. He also constructed a bomb calorimeter in which he measured the heats of combustion of various proteins, fats, and carbohydrates, and of the organic material in the urine and feces, and so arrived at factors for calculating the caloric value of foods to man. Voit measured the amounts of food that people ate and calculated what these amounted to in terms of protein, fat, carbohydrate, and energy. Pettenkoffer and Voit, in Munich, constructed a chamber in which a man could live for several days while his consumption of oxygen and output of carbon dioxide could be measured. Atwater spent some time in Germany as a pupil of both Voit and Rubner at the end of the 19th Century, and when he returned to the United States in 1892, to the Storrs Agriculture Experiment Station, Connecticut, he immediately began building and improving on what he had learned in Germany. He and a physicist, Rosa, constructed a calorimeter large enough for a man to live inside for several days and to take some exercise on a stationary bicycle. With this apparatus Atwater and Benedict (1) showed that the available energy pro-

1

vided by the food eaten by the individual equaled the energy lost by him as heat. In other words, the law of conservation of energy held for man, and it is difficult to overestimate the importance of this discovery. Atwater (2) made a study of the digestibility and availability of protein, fat, and carbohydrate in the diet of man, and Atwater and Bryant (3) revised Rubner's factors for calculating the energy a man derives from these nutrients in his diet.

One of Atwater's practical contributions to knowledge was the compilation of the chemical composition of American food materials, first published in 1896 with C. D. Woods, and revised with A. P. Bryant in 1906 (4). Atwater measured the food intakes of persons, usually men, in many walks of life, and expressed them in terms of protein, fat, carbohydrate, and energy. Using average figures, he demonstrated the effect that a man's occupation might have on his food consumption, and consequently energy intake, and claimed that heavy manual workers such as lumbermen might take up to 8000 kcal a day.

In Chapter 6 Dr. Pi-Sunyer will discuss energy metabolism and obesity. Obesity was not recognized as a serious nutritional problem until the second half of this century, and during the first five decades people were concerned with undernutrition and too little food rather than with overnutrition and too much. Two world wars and the years of depression between them served to emphasize this, and during World War II Dr. Ancel Keys and his colleagues at the University of Minnesota tackled the problem experimentally. Thirty-two young men were deprived of sufficient food and of calories for 6 months, and they were then rehabilitated for 12 weeks. The food during the period of semistarvation provided 1570 calories a day, about half the normal intake. Thousands of measurements were made on the subjects throughout the study, and as you know the whole investigation is described in detail in two large volumes entitled *The Biology of Human Starvation* (5).

In 1946 we went to Germany to study the effects of a shortage of food on a civilian population. Our work complemented that of Keys and co-workers in that the American investigators made a controlled experiment, and were able to study their subjects on the way down as well as during rehabilitation on the way up, while we took the situation as we found it. We studied the effects of undernutrition on various systems of the body, and we also followed some undernourished men, old and young, some of them prisoners who had returned from Russia, while we provided them with unlimited food. Our results were published as a Medical Research Council Special Report (6).

VITAMINS

Now let us go back to the year 1906 when Atwater completed his work. Just about then Hopkins, in the Physiological Laboratory at Cambridge, was making some experiments that were to revolutionize all the current ideas about food and nutrition. Although Hopkins is generally regarded as the discoverer of the vitamins, he was only one in a long line of investigators who contributed to the final understanding of the importance of accessory food factors for life and health. The earliest observations were clinical ones. Scurvy had been a menace to seamen ever since long voyages had been undertaken and, although it was known that it could be prevented by some fresh food, and in 1774 Captain Cook did successfully prevent it in this way, Captain Scott was allowed to leave for the Antarctic without any precautions to avoid scurvy, and sadly scurvy sealed the fate of the party that reached the South Pole in 1911.

Pellagra became a disease of note in the early 18th Century when maize was introduced as a dietary staple and poor people in various parts of the world began to live on little else. Beriberi was a disease generated technologically when rice began to be milled to produce the preferred white variety. The explorer, doctor, and missionary David Livingstone recorded lesions of the eyes of Africans which we now call xerophthalmia. Rickets, the English disease, has probably the longest written history of all vitamin deficiency diseases, for it was first described by Whistler in 1645, but the best known early description was written by Glisson in 1650. Cod liver oil was used to cure it in Scotland and Scandinavia at least as early as the 18th Century.

In spite of all this clinical knowledge, however, disease at the beginning of the 20th Century was still pictured as being caused by an invasion of the body by toxic substances or microbes, and it was very difficult for people to grasp the fact that serious diseases could be due to the absence of minute amounts of some totally unknown substance. It was the use of experimental animals early in the present century that provided the first real advance in the understanding that this could be so. In fact as early as 1881 an animal experiment had been made in Germany, when Lunin showed that mice could not thrive on a diet of casein, butter, fat, and sugar even when supplemented with minerals (7). Hopkins, however, was the one who first grasped the great physiological principle and boldly stated that "No animal can live upon a mixture of pure protein, fat, and carbohydrate, and even when the necessary inorganic material is carefully supplied the animal still cannot flourish. The animal body is adjusted to live either upon plant tissues or the tissues of other animals, and these contain countless substances other than proteins, carbohydrates, and fats. Physiological evolution, I believe, has made some of these well-nigh as essential as are the basal constituents of the diet" (8).

Now what did Hopkins actually do? In the first place he used rats as his experimental animals. This was a new idea at the time—the favorite animal of the German investigators at the end of the last century had been the dog. So novel was the use of the rat and so little did Hopkins know about rats that he was surprised to discover that the males grew faster than the females (9). He had groups of 4 to 6 animals weighing 30–50 g. He fed them all on a diet consisting of 22% casein, 42% raw potato starch, 21% cane sugar, 12–13% lard, and 2–3% of mineral salts produced by incinerating equal parts of oats and dog biscuits. He stated specifically that he provided no roughage. To one group of animals in each experiment he gave fresh milk, 1, 2, or 3 mL per rat per day. Those having milk grew, and the more milk they had the faster the gain in weight. Those not having milk ate less food and failed to grow and soon began to lose weight, so that after about 20 days the experiment had to be terminated. If after 18 days the treatment was reversed, those now given milk started to grow, while those deprived of milk lost weight. Thus it was postulated that the milk contained something that was essential for growth and health of the animals. So far so good. But although this discovery sparked off a tremendous amount of work, which we shall come back to in a minute, I should like first to continue the story as it concerns Hopkins. Nobody could repeat his original experiments. Thirty years later, therefore, he decided to repeat them himself (10). I well remember going to his laboratory in the early 1940s and his telling me about this. The reason nobody could repeat his work was the usual one; nobody had done *exactly* what he did, and part of the trouble was that he did not describe in his original paper every experimental detail of his procedure. It appeared that it was essential to use raw potato starch as the main source of carbohydrate. Raw potato starch is not as well digested as other forms of raw starch, or cooked starch, or sugar. Undigested potato starch reaches the cecum where it ferments, causes the cecum to enlarge and the cecal contents have an acid pH, and it also results in the synthesis of B vitamins, which are then absorbed (11). However, anyone following what Hopkins said he did in his original experiments could not have got the results he got for they would have found that the rats grew splendidly whether they had milk or not. In fact he shows this in his later paper (10). One thing was done in the original experiments which was not mentioned in the paper, except to say that it was not done, and this was to give the animals roughage in the form of strips of filter paper dipped in a weak sugar solution before they were fed. I wonder if Hopkins even knew about this—it may have been a bit of enterprise on the part of his animal technician. Be that as it may, the filter paper prevented refection, prevented synthesis of B vitamins in the cecum, the animals became deficient in B vitamins, and the small quantities of milk given them must have been just sufficient enough for their needs, although it is difficult to see how such small amounts of milk could have done so.

Now let us go back to 1907 and the story of vitamin C. Holst and Frölich were working at the University of Christiania, now Oslo, and by good fortune they used guinea pigs as their experimental animals. When these animals were fed on cereals, without any fresh vegetable food, they developed a disease that corresponded to human scurvy. When the diet contained fresh cabbage or potatoes the disease did not occur. Holst and Frölich (12) made the further observation that the "nutriment" they postulated these fresh foods contained was partially, though not entirely, lost by boiling the cabbage in water for half an hour. This work did not receive the attention it should have at the time, though their paper preceded Hopkins's full publication by 5 years. Twenty-one years later Szent-Györgyi (13), a Hungarian who had worked in Hopkins's laboratory at Cambridge and was interested in reducing substances in biological materials, isolated an acid from cabbage and adrenal cortex which he called hexuronic acid because the molecule had six carbon atoms. Svirbely and Szent-Györgyi (14) showed that this substance, extracted from ox suprarenal glands, protected guinea pigs against scurvy. Dr. Glen King also spent some time in "Hoppy's" department, and in 1932 King and Waugh (15) and Waugh and King (16) isolated vitamin C from lemon juice and identified it with Szent-Györgyi's hexuronic acid. In 1933 the structural formula of vitamin C was established (17, 18), and later in the same year Reichstein and colleagues in Switzerland (19) and workers in Haworth's laboratory in Liverpool (20) synthesized it.

In 1912, when Hopkins's main paper was published, Osborne and Mendel (21) were working at Yale, and they were convinced by his work of the special nutritive value of milk for rats, so they tested its various constituents. They found that butter fat, and also cod liver oil, had much greater growth promoting properties for the rat than lard. McCollum and Davis (22), then in Wisconsin, also using rats, tried various fats to supplement cereal diets and found that butter fat and egg yolk promoted growth, but lard did not. Even butter fat, however, was ineffective when the rest of the diet consisted of polished rice, casein, and minerals, but it was found that a supplement of wheat germ enabled the animals to grow. This gave McCollum and Davis (23) the clue that two factors, fat soluble A and water soluble B, were necessary for the growth of their experimental animals. McCollum and Simmonds (24) realized that the fat soluble A factor had functions other than promoting growth. Deficiency of the fat soluble A factor produced eye lesions, and McCollum and Simmonds introduced the word xerophthalmia to describe this condition. McCollum therefore was the first to realize that there were at least two accessory food factors, one soluble in fat, the other in water. I did not meet McCollum until 1936 when, as a young and inexperienced research worker, I visited his laboratory at Johns Hopkins. He was a great man, yet he treated me with courtesy and kindness, and made me feel as though I was someone who mattered, and I have never forgotten this lesson and example. But this is by the way. To Bloch (25) in Copenhagen goes the credit of demonstrating that xerophthalmia in young children was caused by feeding them on milk from which the fat had been removed, and concoctions of flour. The disease, if recognized in time, could be cured with cod liver oil, but whole milk, butter, cream, and eggs contained the curative factor in small quantities.

At this time, that is, around 1920, investigators could not help noticing that the fats and foods containing the fat soluble factor were yellow, and the idea that yellowness was associated with the factor was strengthened when McCollum, Simmonds, and Pitz (26) and Osborne and Mendel (27) showed that green vegetables, known to contain yellow pigments carotene and xanthophyll, were effective as a source of fat soluble A, and Steenbock (28) demonstrated that carotene was the active pigment.

The subsequent history of vitamin A during the first 50 years of this century—the understanding of the relationship between carotene and vitamin A, the appreciation of the necessity of vitamin A for a healthy skin as well as its vital importance for the eye, and the working out of its structural formula and subsequent synthesis—is too long for me to go into in detail. I would refer those interested to Moore's excellent book (29).

Going back now to 1914, members of the Medical Research Committee in England, as it was then called, realized that rickets was still a great scourge in Britain and they invited Edward Mellanby to look into it. Mellanby knew that puppies got rickets, so he decided to use them as his experimental animals. He found they got rickets if they were fed on a diet of cereals and milk, and he concluded that rickets is primarily due to the lack of an accessory food factor in the diet (30, 31). At first he thought this was McCollum's fat soluble A, but further work (32) led him to believe that two unknown factors were involved because some fats were effective in curing lesions of the eyes and others in curing rickets. Cod liver oil would cure both.

Meanwhile another form of treatment was on the way. Fresh air and exercise had long been recognized as preventing rickets, and in 1890 Palm (33) had emphasized the importance of sunlight. After the end of World War I in 1918, Dr. Harriette Chick and some colleagues from the Lister Institute in London went to von Pirquet's clinic in Vienna and showed by controlled experiments that exposure to sunlight cured rickets as well as did the administration of cod liver oil. Their reports were published in 1922 and 1923 (34, 35). Huldschinsky (36) showed that light from a mercury vapor lamp was effective, and this was confirmed by Chick et al. (35). Our understanding of how sunlight acts on the provitamin 7 dehydrocholesterol in the skin to form vitamin D_3, calciferol, and the similar action of ultraviolet light on ergosterol in plants to form vitamin D_2, was the result of many workers' efforts, but the paper by Hume and Smith (37) is one of the most important ones. Margot Hume and Hannah Henderson Smith, a nursing sister, had both participated in the work in Vienna. In later years I came to know Dr. Chick, Dr. Hume, and Sister Smith quite well, and Dame Harriette Chick and Dr. Hume often came to visit us when we were working in Germany after World War II, as indeed did Sir Edward and Lady Mellanby.

My acquaintance with Mellanby dates from the 1930s, by which time he was Secretary of the Medical Research Council. In his experiments on puppies he had found that, although rickets was due primarily to the deficiency of a fat soluble factor, some cereals had a rickets-producing effect on a marginally vitamin D deficient diet. Oatmeal was particularly bad, but the effect could be counteracted by adding calcium carbonate to the diet. Mellanby postulated that whole cereals contained a positive anticalcifying agent, or toxamin (38). Not everybody agreed with him, and in 1937 the American Medical Association Council on Foods (39) agreed that "It may be concluded that there is no good evidence for the existence of a decalcifying factor in cereals, and that the hypothesis of the existence of such a factor is not needed to explain the experimental results." Mellanby was right, of course, and in 1939 he and Harrison (40) demonstrated that the anticalcifying agent was phytic acid, which is present combined with potassium and magnesium in whole cereals; the calcium salt is less soluble, so calcium from the rest of the diet is precipitated in the intestine and its absorption prevented. Harrison and Mellanby (40) made their experiments on puppies, and we followed this up by demonstrating that the same thing was true for man (41, 42).

The story of how the B vitamins were sorted out is also a long one. In 1911 Funk (43) had obtained a concentrate from rice polishings which cured polyneuritis in pigeons. Funk coined the word vitamine, later changed to vitamin when it was realized that accessory food factors were not all organic bases.

Pure vitamin B_1 was isolated from rice polishings by Jansen and Donath (44) and shown by Peters and his colleagues at Oxford in 1929 to form part of an enzyme system involved in carbohydrate metablism (45). The structural formula was determined by Windaus and collaborators in Germany in 1932 (46) and synthesized by Williams and Cline in the United States in 1936 (47).

Until 1926 it had been generally believed that vitamin B was a single substance, but in that year Smith and Hendrick (48) in the United States showed that it consisted of at least two water soluble factors. One, which prevented and cured beriberi, was thermolabile; the other, present in brewer's yeast, was thermostable and was essential for the growth of experimental animals.

A disease of prisoners in Nyasaland had been described by Stannus in 1912 and 1913 (49, 50); it involved soreness of the tongue and lips, and angles of the mouth (later called angular stomatitis). Stannus thought this was pellagra, though the diet consisted largely of rice, not maize. In 1925 Goldberger and Tanner (51) showed that the disease, which they also thought was pellagra, was cured by yeast.

In 1932 Warburg and Christian in Germany discovered what they called the yellow enzyme, which had growth-promoting properties (52), and in 1933 Kuhn in Germany (53) and Karrer and colleagues in Switzerland (54) synthesized riboflavin. The relation between this substance and the clinical symptoms originally described by Stannus was established in 1938 by Dr. Sebrell when he described the production of riboflavin deficiency in dogs (55), and in man (56).

The history of pellagra goes back to the 18th Century. The disease is characterized by a dermatitis, accentuated by light, which means that the cheeks, the front of the neck, and the backs of the hands suffer most, and the mouth and tongue are often sore. Severe cases may become demented. It was appreciated that pellagra occurred among poor people who ate maize as their staple food and it was widespread in Europe, particularly in Italy and Spain, and also in the Ukraine and Egypt. The disease must have been endemic in the Southern United States, but was brought to the fore by the poverty following the Civil War in the 19th Century. Nicotinic acid, β pyridine carboxylic acid, was known as a chemical compound and to be a constituent of foodstuffs, particularly of yeast, many years before its relation to pellagra was discovered. In 1937 a disease of dogs, known as black tongue, which is similar to human pellagra in many ways, was found by Elvehjem and his colleagues to be cured by nicotinic acid (57). As soon as Elvehjem's paper was published, several groups of workers gave nicotinic acid to patients with pellagra, also with beneficial results (58–60). There still remained the puzzle as to why pellagra should be confined to maize-eating populations, since maize contains as much nicotinic acid as wheat and rice. This was not solved until after 1950, so I must leave that part of the story.

I have no time to speak in detail about the other B vitamins. Suffice it to say that by 1950 pyridoxine, biotin, pantothenic acid, and folic acid had all been synthesized and their activities characterized. In 1948 vitamin B_{12}, whose molecule is the most complex of all the vitamins, was isolated almost simultaneously in the United States by Rickes et al. (61), and in Britain by Lester-Smith and Parker (62) and shown to be active in the treatment of pernicious anemia (63).

TRACE ELEMENTS

In Chapter 3 Dr. Sandstead will discuss trace elements, and I think he will agree that Underwood is the name above all others that we associate with these dietary essentials. Underwood's book *Trace Elements in Human and Animal Nutrition,* first published in 1956 (64), with a third edition in 1971 (65), is a classic. However, Underwood, who worked in Australia, was not the original discoverer of the importance of trace elements in nutrition. He makes this abundantly clear in his book and in an unfinished article he wrote shortly before his death in 1980 which was to have been presented at a meeting organized by the Royal Society and held in London in January 1981 (66). Underwood's contribution was his extensive knowledge of the subject as a whole.

The trace elements with the longest history are iodine and iron. In fact, the story of both goes back at least 2000 years to the Greeks, who were reputed to have used burnt sponges to cure goiter and drinking water in which a sword had been allowed to rust to treat anemia. These treatments were quite empirical, and it was not until the 19th Century that the relationship between iodine and goiter and between iron and anemia was realized. In both instances the original observations were made on man and the functions of the elements in the body were worked out in man, without the use of experimental animals so widely used for research on other trace elements.

The observation that iodine cured goiter and the suggestion that goiter might be caused by a deficiency of iodine, were made by French physicians in the early 1890s. By the end of the 19th Century it had been shown that iodine was concentrated in the thyroid gland, and that the concentration in goitrous glands was low. In 1919 Kendall (67) isolated a crystalline compound from the thyroid containing 65% iodine, which he named thyroxine, and in 1927 Harington and Barger (68) showed that thyroxine was a compound of phenol and tyrosine containing four iodine atoms in the molecule, and they were able to synthesize it.

By the 18th Century it was known that blood contains iron, and it was thought that the iron was confined to the globular part. In the early part of the 19th Century methods were developed for the measurement of hemoglobin and of iron in blood. These methods were inaccurate by present-day standards, but they served to show that the concentration of iron and of hemoglobin in the blood of anemic women was low and that it could be raised by giving a medicinal iron salt.

By the early years of this century the role of hemoglobin in oxygen transport had been described. Then in the 1920s Keilin and his co-workers demonstrated that iron had other functions in the body, and that as part of the cytochrome enzymes it was concerned in the oxidative mechanisms of all living cells. Meanwhile Abderhalden and Bunge in Germany had been studying the amounts of iron in foods, and in the

livers of animals of different ages, and the amounts absorbed and excreted. Since the feces always contain iron it was assumed that the intestine actively excreted as well as absorbed it. Then in 1937 we published a
paper that challenged this idea (69). It all started with a patient, Mrs.
Harris, who was suffering from polycythemia rubra vera. This disease is
characterized by far too many red blood cells, and consequently very
sticky blood. One treatment was to give a drug called phenylhydrazine.
This drug causes breakdown of the red cells and when this happens the
iron in the hemoglobin in the red cells is set free inside the body. We
reckoned that Mrs. Harris had about twice as much iron in her body as a
normal person, 10 g instead of 5 g. We measured the amount of iron in
Mrs. Harris's food and drink, and in her urine and feces while she was
having the drug. We fully expected Mrs. Harris to excrete far more iron
than she took in in her food as the drug took effect, but to our astonish-
ment almost all the 5 g or so of iron from the broken down red cells
stayed inside her body and virtually none was excreted. We then looked
carefully at the literature on the absorption and excretion of iron and we
came to the conclusion that practically no iron is excreted either by the
intestine or by the kidneys, and that the amount of iron in the body is
maintained by controlled absorption. We put this idea to the test by in-
jecting intravenously into ourselves and our friends measured amounts
of an iron salt every day for 14 days, and following our intakes and ex-
cretions of iron while we were doing so. Again we found that very little
of the iron injected was excreted (70). So our hypothesis seemed to be
correct (71), and it has been proved to be so many times since. A lot of
work followed in America to discover how this controlled absorption is
achieved, particularly by Hahn and his co-workers (72) and Granick
(73), and the mucosal block theory was proposed. The use of radioactive
isotopes is throwing more light on this problem.

Copper was the next element to be recognized as essential for life, and
the credit for this discovery goes to Hart and co-workers (74) in
Wisconsin. They showed that copper as well as iron was necessary for
blood formation in rats. They were the first to master the technique of
feeding rats purified diets containing all known essential minerals apart
from the one they were studying, and within a few years they had used
this technique to show that manganese and zinc were also essential elements for mice and rats (75, 76), and Orent and McCollum (77) demonstrated the importance of manganese to the functioning of the sexual
organs.

During the 1930s interest in trace elements broadened because it was realized that naturally occurring disorders in man and in domestic animals were caused by deficient or excessive intakes of trace elements other than iodine and iron. From America and North Africa came reports of the effects of excess fluoride from industrial fumes and dusts which had contaminated the grass and water supply, causing disordered bones and teeth in man and animals (78, 79). The appreciation that too much fluorine caused mottled enamel of the teeth and lesions of the bones came about 10 years before it was realized that too little fluorine predisposed children to dental caries (80).

In 1935 two papers were published describing debilitating diseases of sheep and cattle in Australia, called "coast disease" or "wasting disease" (81, 82). This disease was shown to be due to cobalt deficiency. The relation between cobalt and vitamin B_{12} was not then appreciated and it was not until 1948, when the antipernicious factor in liver was discovered to contain cobalt (83), and the full explanation of this deficiency disease was understood. Monogastric animals, including man, cannot synthesize vitamin B_{12} and their only requirement for cobalt is as the vitamin B_{12} molecule. Ruminants, however, do synthesize vitamin B_{12} in the rumen, but in order to do so they must have cobalt, and the cattle and sheep with coast disease were in fact suffering from vitamin B_{12} deficiency.

Toxic intakes of trace elements as well as deficiencies have also caused serious problems in livestock, particularly in cattle and sheep. Copper poisoning, with hemolysis of the red cells and hemoglobinuria, was reported from many parts of the world from the 1930s onward (65). This led to the appreciation that the trace elements interact with one another and that an excess of one might predispose to a deficiency of another. For example, high intakes of molybdenum increase the likelihood of signs of copper deficiency when the copper intake is moderately low. When the copper intake is very high molybdenum can prevent signs of toxicity, and additional iron and zinc have a similar effect. The mechanisms of these interactions were worked out after 1950 and therefore come outside the period of history that has been assigned to me.

NUTRITION, PHYSICAL GROWTH, AND MENTAL DEVELOPMENT

This is the topic of Dr. Winick's chapter. It is true there have been advances in the last 30 years, particularly as regards mental development, but anyone who wants to know anything about the history of the study of human growth will find everything he needs in a book by Tanner published in 1981 (84). The study of physical growth started long before 1900, and investigators in the first 50 years of this century were building on the experience of those that had gone before. Thus, the effect of poverty and illness on physical growth was already appreciated in the 19th Century. At that time Europe was still in the forefront of medical and scientific research, and measurements of height and weight of school children from different backgrounds were made in Italy, Denmark, Sweden, Germany, France, and Britain. Important studies were also starting in America, and that of Porter in St. Louis was outstanding (85). Porter had worked in Germany and, like Atwater, he built on his experiences there. He was the first to relate body size to mental ability at school, and this relationship was recorded by subsequent American investigators. Much of the work during the first 50 years of this century was directed to the production of standards for growth. The shortcomings of cross-sectional, as compared with longitudinal, measurements came to be appreciated, particularly over the period of rapid growth associated with puberty. Since this occurs at different ages in individual children cross-sectional studies always mask the changes that can be expected in the growth of an individual child. The United States led the way in longitudinal growth studies and the work of Baldwin in New York and Chicago (86), and later in Iowa (87) pioneered the way. The Harvard Growth Study (88) was particularly important because the data were so fully analyzed, and the value of expressing growth in terms of increments rather than status was emphasized for the first time. Increments show the effect of immediate environmental alterations, including those of nutrition.

By the 1920s it was generally agreed that poor nutrition led to poor growth (89), and 1926 saw the publication in Britain of a report by Corry Mann (90) describing the effects of equicalorific amounts of milk, butter, sugar, or margarine on the growth of children in one of Dr. Barnado's homes in the south of England. The children receiving the milk (1 (English) pint a day) grew better than any of the others and this led to the idea, already foreshadowed by Hopkins's discovery, that there was something special about milk for the growth and health of schoolchildren. In Britain this was followed by a number of investigations all purporting to demonstrate this almost magical value of milk. However, few of these studies were properly controlled, and the control group generally had no supplement or only a placebo. Many other foods might have given just as good a response as milk, and all that can be said with certainty is that the various basal diets must have been unappetizing or nutritionally unsatisfactory. We found when we were working in Germany between 1946 and 1949 that a supplement of milk given to children who were already receiving adequate calories, protein, calcium, and vitamin D made no difference to the growth rate, even though 75% of the energy in the basal diet was derived from bread (91).

NUTRITION AND PREGNANCY

Dr. Rosso will discuss newer concepts about nutrition and pregnancy. I am concerned with the older work and one of the earliest systematic attempts to determine the effect of nutrition on the size of the baby at birth was made by Smith in 1916 (92). He analyzed records from London and Dublin hospitals and concluded that a poor state of nutrition increased the likelihood of a woman's having a dead or a premature baby, and that the average weight of full term babies born to poorly nourished mothers was slightly less than that of babies born to better nourished ones.

There were food shortages during and after World War I and papers were published concerning the size of the babies born during this time. Many of these papers, however, were inconclusive and even contradictory. In the summary given by Krogman (93) there were 29 references to authors who reported that infants born during the war were smaller than normal, and 26 to other authors who found no such effect. In the period between the wars studies were made to find out the effects of the inadequate diets of poor women in various parts of the world. These were reviewed by Garry and Stiven (94) and Garry and Wood (95). The general conclusion was that the weights of children born to mothers at the lower end of the socioeconomic scale were usually a little below the average for those in families better off financially, and that poor nutrition was probably one of the causes. There were some studies in which poorly nourished women were given food supplements during pregnancy. This supplementation appeared to reduce the incidence of still-births and neonatal deaths (96–100).

Just after World War II ended in 1945, Dr. Clement Smith from the Boston Lying-in Hospital, went to the Netherlands to find out what he could about the effect of the severe shortage of food during the transport strike lasting from September 1944 to May 1945 on the mother and babies. Dr. Smith, like Dame Harriette Chick after World War I, took advantage of a situation that had arisen because of the war to study the effects of severe nutritional deficiency on a vulnerable section of the population. Neither of these studies could have been made in happier times. Dr. Smith came to visit us in Cambridge on his way back from the Netherlands, and I remember so well how he spread out all his data before us and we discussed its implications. He found (101, 102) that there was a sharp fall in the weights of children born in hospitals in The Hague and Rotterdam during the period of hunger if this had occurred in the last 3 or 4 months of pregnancy, and this was in spite of the fact that the pregnant women did get supplementary rations. Recovery was rapid, and by the beginning of July 1945 the birth weights had returned to their prewar level. Smith appreciated that average figures can be midleading and he preferred to express his results as medians or percentiles. In this way he was able to show that weights of large and small infants were reduced by approximately the same percentage, and the weights of infants in the middle range were reduced by 240 g. There was an even more severe food shortage during the siege of Leningrad, which lasted from August 1941 to January 1943, and Antonov (103) described the situation. "On a diet hardly sufficient to keep them alive the women had to undergo physical exertions to which many of them had not been accustomed, such as standing in long lines for bread and other things in the biting cold and often at night, walking long distances, sometimes with heavy loads, chopping wood, clearing snow and ice." Of the infants born during the first half of 1942 over 81% weighed less than 3000 g and the average birth weight was over 500 g less than it had been before the siege.

During our three years in Germany after World War II, Dean (104) analyzed the excellent German records of birth weights in a large maternity hospital in Wuppertal from 1937 through 1948. Before the war, in 1937 and 1938, food was plentiful. Rationing was in force during the war years and there was a slight decline in average birth weight. The time of most severe food shortage came after the war, during 1945, though it was never as extreme as it had been in Leningrad and Holland. In 1945 median birthweight was 150 g less than it had been in prewar years.

Thus these studies and others all showed that the state of nutrition of the mother during pregnancy affected the birth weight of the baby and the more severe the undernutrition the greater the effect. Studies on animals produced similar conclusions (105, 106).

NUTRITION AND IMMUNITY

During the first 50 years of this century surprisingly little work was published on the ability of the undernourished person to produce antibodies, in spite of the widely held belief that famine and starvation is an important cause of epidemics. Dr. Gell came to Germany with us in 1946 and he was one of the first to study this experimentally. Gell used a triple antigen containing a bacterium, a pure protein from tobacco mosaic virus, and fowl erythrocytes for his tests. His conclusion was that in 51 undernourished individuals the response was significantly less than in 16 normally nourished controls. There was, however, no correlation between the amount of weight lost by the undernourished subjects and the concentration of proteins in their serum (107).

SUBJECTS FOR THE FUTURE

The subjects for the future I shall not discuss, for there is little to say about their progress in the first 50 years of this century. Suffice it to say that they relate to current problems concerning man, and as such must be investigated in man. Studies with human beings are difficult and generally laborious, but over the first 50 years of this century, from Atwater's time onward, investigators have been willing to make them, often using themselves as subjects, with important if not always spectacular results. Studies on animals, however, have also played their part. It is doubtful whether Hopkins would ever have been able to postulate the existence of accessory food factors had he not chosen to use a fast-growing animal like the rat, and certain that Holst and Frölich would not have discovered the existence of vitamin C had they not elected to use guinea pigs. The wise French physician and experimentalist Claude Bernard realized this in the middle of the 19th Century when he wrote "Le choix intelligent d'un animal présentant une disposition anatomique heureuse est souvent la condition essentielle du succès d'une expérience et de la solution d'un problème physiologique très important" (108).

REFERENCES

1. W. O. Atwater and F. G. Benedict, "Experiments on the Metabolism of Matter and Energy in the Human Body," *U.S. Dept. Agriculture Bull. No. 69*, Washington D.C., 1899.

2. W. O. Atwater, "On the Digestibility and Availability of Food Materials," *Conn. (Storrs) Agricultural Exp. Sta. 14th Ann. Report*, 1901.

3. W. O. Atwater and A. P. Bryant, "The Availability and Fuel Value of Food Materials," *Conn. (Storrs) Agricultural Exp. Sta. 12th Ann. Report*, 1899.

4. W. O. Atwater and A. P. Bryant, "The Chemical Composition of American Food Materials," *U.S. Dept. Agriculture Office of Experiment Stations Bull. No. 28*, (Revised), 1906.

5. A. Keys, J. Brožek, A. Henschel, O. Mickelsen, and H. L. Taylor, *The Biology of Human Starvation*, Minneapolis, University of Minnesota Press, 1950.

6. Members of the Department of Experimental Medicine, Cambridge, and Associated Workers, *Studies of Undernutrition, Wuppertal 1946-9*, Spec. Rep. Ser. Med. Res. Coun. No. 275, HMSO, London, 1951.

7. G. Lunin, *Z. Physiol. Chem.*, **5**, 31 (1881).

8. F. G. Hopkins, *Analyst*, **31**, 395 (1906).

9. F. G. Hopkins, *J. Physiol.*, **44**, 425 (1912).

10. F. G. Hopkins and V. R. Leader, *J. Hygiene*, **44**, 149 (1945).

11. P. M. Kon, S. K. Kon, and T. R. Mattick, *J. Hygiene*, **38**, 1 (1938).

12. A. Holst and T. Frölich, *J. Hygiene*, **7**, 634 (1907).

13. A. Szent-Györgyi, *Biochem. J.*, **22**, 1387 (1928).

14. J. L. Svirbely and A. Szent-Györgyi, *Biochem. J.*, **26**, 865 (1932).

15. C. G. King and W. A. Waugh, *Science*, **75**, 357 (1932).

16. W. A. Waugh and C. G. King, *J. Biol. Chem.*, **97**, 325 (1932).

17. R. W. Herbert, E. G. V. Percival, R. J. W. Reynolds, F. Smith, and E. L. Hirst, *J. Soc. Chem. Ind.*, **52**, 221 and 481 (1933).

18. P. Karrer, K. Schoof, and F. Zehender, *Helv. Chim. Acta*, **16**, 1161 (1933).

19. T. Reichstein, A. Grussner, and R. Oppenauer, *Helv. Chim. Acta*, **16**, 1019 (1933).

20. R. G. Ault, D. K. Baird, H. C. Carrington, W. N. Haworth, R. W. Herbert, E. L. Hirst, E. G. V. Percival, F. Smith, and M. Stacey, *J. Chem. Soc.*, **2**, 1419 (1933).

21. T. B. Osborne and L. B. Mendel, *J. Biol. Chem.*, **15**, 311 (1913).

22. E. V. McCollum and M. Davis, *J. Biol. Chem.*, **15**, 167 (1913).

23. E. V. McCollum and M. Davis, *J. Biol. Chem.*, **23**, 181 (1915).

24. E. V. McCollum and N. Simmonds, *J. Biol. Chem.*, **32**, 181 (1917).

25. C. E. Bloch, *J. Hygiene*, **19**, 283 (1921).

26. E. V. McCollum, N. Simmonds, and W. Pitz, *J. Biol. Chem.*, **30**, 13 (1917).

27. T. B. Osborne and L. B. Mendel, *J. Biol. Chem.*, **37**, 187 (1919).

28. H. Steenbock, *Science*, **50**, 352 (1919).

29. T. Moore, *Vitamin A*, Amsterdam, Elsevier, 1957.

30. E. Mellanby, *J. Physiol.*, **52**, Proceedings xi–xii (1918).

31. E. Mellanby, *J. Physiol.*, **52**, Proceedings liii–liv (1918).

32. E. Mellanby, *Lancet*, **1**, 856 (1920).

33. T. A. Palm, *Practitioner*, **14**, 270 and 321 (1890).

34. H. Chick, E. J. Dalyell, M. Hume, H. M. M. Mackay, H. Henderson-Smith, and H. Wimberger, *Lancet*, **2**, 7 (1922).

35. H. Chick, E. J. Dalyell, E. M. Hume, H. M. M. Mackay, H. H. Smith, and H. Wimberger, *Studies of Rickets in Vienna 1919-1922*, Spec. Rep. Ser. Med. Res. Coun. No. 77, HMSO, London, 1923.

36. K. Huldschinsky, *Deutsche Med. Woch.*, **45**, 712 (1919).

37. E. M. Hume and H. H. Smith, *Biochem. J.*, **18**, 1334 (1924).

38. E. Mellanby, *J. Physiol.*, **61**, XXIVP-XXVIP (1926).

39. American Medical Association Council on Foods, *J.A.M.A.*, **109**, 30 (1937).

40. D. C. Harrison and E. Mellanby, *Biochem. J.*, **33**, 1660 (1939).

41. R. A. McCance and E. M. Widdowson, *J. Physiol.*, **101**, 44 (1942).

42. R. A. McCance and E. M. Widdowson, *J. Physiol.*, **101**, 304 (1942).

43. C. Funk, *J. Physiol.*, **43**, 395 (1911).

44. B. P. C. Jansen and W. F. Donath, *Chem. Weekblad.*, **23**, 201 (1926).

45. H. W. Kinnersley and R. A. Peters, *Biochem. J.*, **23**, 1126 (1929).

46. A. Windaus, R. Tschesche, and H. Ruhkopf, *Nach. v. der. Ges. Wiss. Göttingen, III*, 207 (1932).

47. R. R. Williams and J. K. Cline, *J. Am. Chem. Soc.*, **58**, 1504 (1936).

48. M. I. Smith and E. G. Hendrick, *Pub. Health Rep. Washington*, **41**, 201 (1926).

49. H. Stannus, *Trans. Soc. Trop. Med. Hyg.*, **5**, 112 (1912).

50. H. Stannus, *Trans. Soc. Trop. Med. Hyg.*, **7**, 32 (1913).

51. J. Goldberger and W. F. Tanner, *Public Health Reports*, **40**, 54 (1925).

52. O. Warburg and W. Christian, *Biochem. Z.*, **254**, 438 (1932).

53. R. Kuhn, K. Reinemund, F. Weygand, and R. Ströbele, *Ber. Deutsch. Chem. Gesellsch.*, **68**, 1765 (1935).

54. P. Karrer, B. Becker, F. Benz, P. Frei, H. Salomon, and K. Schöpp, *Helv. Chim. Acta*, **18**, 1435 (1935).

55. W. H. Sebrell and R. H. Onstott, *Pub. Health. Rep. U.S. Treas. Dept.*, **53**, 83 (1938).

56. W. B. Sebrell and R. E. Butler, *Pub. Health Rep. Washington*, **53**, 2282 (1938).

57. C. A. Elvehjem, R. J. Madden, F. M. Strong, and D. W. Wooley, *J. Am. Chem. Soc.*, **59**, 1767 (1937).

58. T. D. Spies, C. Cooper, and M. A. Blankerhorn, *J.A.M.A.*, **110**, 622 (1938).

59. T. D. Spies, J. M. Grant, R. E. Stone, and J. B. McLester, *Southern Med. J.*, **31**, 1231 (1938).

60. V. P. Sydenstricker, H. L. Schmidt, M. C. Fulton, J. C. New, and L. Geeslin, *Southern Med. J.*, **31**, 1155 (1938).

61. E. L. Rickes, N. G. Brink, F. R. Koniuszy, T. R. Wood, and K. Folkers, *Science*, **107**, 396 (1948).

62. E. Lester-Smith and L. F. J. Parker, *Biochem. J.*, **43**, iii-ix (1948).

63. R. West, *Science*, **107**, 398 (1948).

64. E. J. Underwood, *Trace Elements in Human and Animal Nutrition*, 1st ed., New York, Academic, 1956.

65. E. J. Underwood, *Trace Elements in Human and Animal Nutrition*, 3rd ed., New York, Academic, 1971.

66. E. J. Underwood, *Phil. Trans. R. Soc. Lond. B*, **294**, 3 (1981).

67. E. C. Kendall, *J. Biol. Chem.*, **39**, 125 (1919).

68. C. R. Harington and G. Barger, *Biochem. J.*, **21**, 169 (1927).

69. R. A. McCance and E. M. Widdowson, *Q. J. Med. N.S.*, **6**, 277 (1937).

70. R. A. McCance and E. M. Widdowson, *J. Physiol.*, **94**, 148 (1938).

71. R. A. McCance and E. M. Widdowson, *Lancet*, **2**, 680 (1937).

72. P. F. Hahn, W. F. Bale, J. F. Ross, W. M. Balfour, and G. H. Whipple, *J. Exp. Med.*, **78**, 169 (1943).

73. S. Granick, *J. Biol. Chem.*, **164**, 737 (1946).

74. E. B. Hart, H. Steenbock, J. Waddell, and C. A. Elvehjem, *J. Biol. Chem.*, **77**, 797 (1928).

75. A. R. Kemmerer, C. A. Elvehjem, and E. B. Hart, *J. Biol. Chem.*, **92**, 623 (1931).

76. W. R. Todd, C. A. Elvehjem, and E. B. Hart, *Am. J. Physiol.*, **107**, 146 (1934).

77. E. R. Orent and E. V. McCollum, *J. Biol. Chem.*, **92**, 651 (1931).

78. H. N. Churchill, *Ind. Eng. Chem.*, **23**, 996 (1931).

79. H. Velu, *C.R. Soc. Biol., Paris*, **108**, 750 (1931).

80. H. T. Dean, "Fluorine and Dental Health," Am. Assoc. Advance. Sci., Washington, D.C., 1942, pp. 6–11 and 23–31.

81. H. R. Marston, *J. Coun. Sci. Ind. Res. (Aust.)*, **8**, 111 (1935).

82. E. J. Underwood and J. F. Filmer, *Aust. Vet. J.*, **11**, 84 (1935).

83. E. Lester-Smith, *Nature,* **162**, 144 (1948).

84. J. M. Tanner, *A History of the Study of Human Growth*, Cambridge, Cambridge University Press, 1981.

85. W. T. Porter, *Trans. Acad. Sci. St. Louis*, **6**, 161 (1893).

86. B. T. Baldwin, *Physical Growth and School Progress: A Study in Experimental Education*, U.S. Bureau of Education Publication No. 10, USBE, Washington, 1914.

87. B. T. Baldwin and T. D. Wood, *Weight-Height-Age Tables. Tables for Boys and Girls of School Age*, American Child Health Association, New York, 1923.

88. F. K. Shuttleworth, *Child Development*, **5**, 89 (1934).

89. D. N. Paton and L. Findlay, *Poverty, Nutrition and Growth. Studies of Child Life in Cities and Rural Districts of Scotland*, Spec. Rep. Ser. Med. Res. Coun. No. 101. HMSO, London, 1926.

90. H. C. Corry Mann, *Diets for Boys During the School Age*, Spec. Rep. Ser. Med. Res. Coun. No. 105, HMSO, London, 1926.

91. E. M. Widdowson and R. A. McCance, *Studies on the Nutritive Value of Bread and on the Effect of Variations in the Extraction Rate of Flour on the Growth of Undernourished Children*, Spec. Rep. Ser. Med. Res. Coun. No. 287. HMSO, London, 1954.

92. G. F. D. Smith, *Lancet*, **2**, 54 (1916).

93. W. M. Krogman, *Growth of Man*, Vol. XX of *Tabulae Biologicae*, Den Haag, Junk, 1941.

94. R. C. Garry and D. Stiven, *Nutr. Abstr. Rev.*, **5**, 855 (1936).

95. R. C. Garry and H. O. Wood, *Nutr. Abstr. Rev.*, **15**, 591 (1946).

96. A. J. Turner, *Med. J. Australia*, **1,** 490 (1938).

97. J. H. Ebbs, W. A. Scott, and F. F. Tisdall, *J. Nutr.*, **21,** No. 6, Suppl. p. 9, Proc. (1941).

98. J. H. Ebbs, F. F. Tisdall and W. A. Scott, *J. Nutr.*, **22,** 515 (1941).

99. J. H. Ebbs, A. Brown, F. F. Tisdall, W. J. Moyle and M. Bell, *Can. Med. Assn. J.*, **46,** 6 (1942).

100. M. I. Balfour, *Lancet*, **1,** 208 (1944).

101. C. A. Smith, *J. Pediat.*, **30,** 229 (1947).

102. C. A. Smith, *Am. J. Obstet. Gynec.*, **53,** 599 (1947).

103. A. N. Antonov, *J. Pediat.*, **30,** 250 (1947).

104. R. F. A. Dean, "The Size of the Baby at Birth and the Yield of Breast Milk," in *Studies of Undernutrition, Wuppertal 1946-49*, Spec. Rep. Ser. Med. Res. Coun. No. 275, HMSO, London, 1951, pp. 346–378.

105. H. D. King, *Anat. Rec.*, **9,** 213 (1915).

106. L. R. Wallace, *J. Agric. Sci.*, **38,** 93 (1945).

107. P. G. H. Gell, "Serological Responses to Antigenic Stimuli," in *Studies of Undernutrition, Wuppertal 1946-49*, Spec. Rep. Ser. Med. Res. Coun. No. 275, HMSO, London, 1951, pp. 193–203.

108. M. C. Bernard, *Introduction a l'étude de la médecine expérimentale*, Paris, Baillière, 1865.

2

Ascorbic Acid as it Relates to the Metabolism of Drugs and Environmental Agents

V. G. ZANNONI, R. L. SUSICK, and R. C. SMART

Department of Pharmacology, University of Michigan Medical School, Ann Arbor, Michigan

The metabolism of xenobiotics is influenced by a variety of environmental, physiological, and genetic factors. These include age, sex, strain, species, stress, and drug-drug interactions, as well as the nutritional state of the organism (1–4). Many laboratories throughout the world have contributed to our knowledge of the hepatic microsomal mixed function oxygenase system (MFO). This system has a major role in the metabolism of a great variety of foreign compounds. This electron transport system is illustrated in Figure 2-1. The involvement of ascorbic acid in drug and steroid metabolism is well established and its role is of current interest (5–9).

Richards and co-workers in 1941 (10) demonstrated that pentobarbital sleeping time was prolonged in scorbutic guinea pigs compared to normal controls and that this result could be reversed by the administration of vitamin C. Subsequently, Axelrod and co-workers in 1954 (11) showed a significant increase in the plasma half-life of acetanilid, aniline, and antipyrine in animals depleted of the vitamin; replenishing the animals with ascorbic acid returned the half-life to normal. Conney and co-workers in 1961 (12) demonstrated that vitamin C deficient guinea pigs were sensitive to the muscle relaxant zoxazolamine. The increased

---

This research was supported by Grant 23007 from Hoffmann-LaRoche.

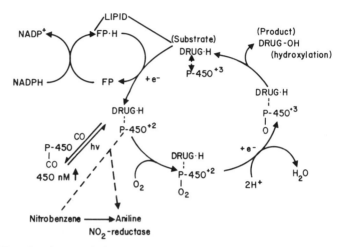

Figure 2-1.   Hepatic microsomal electron transport for drug oxidation and reduction.

duration of this drug in vivo correlated with a decrease in its liver microsomal oxidation in vitro. Degkwitz and Staundinger in 1965 (8) showed that the p-hydroxylation of acetanilid was decreased 90% in vitamin C deficiency and also found that the hydroxylation of coumarin was decreased in deficiency which could be reversed by the in vivo administration of ascorbic acid (9). In 1969 Leber and co-workers (13) demonstrated that liver microsomes from scorbutic animals showed a significant decrease in the demethylation of aminopyrine, hydroxylation of acetanilid, and quantity of cytochrome P-450. Kato and co-workers (14) studied the metabolism of a number of compounds, including aniline, hexobarbital, zoxazolamine, aminopyrine, diphenyhydramine, meperidine, p-nitrobenzoic acid, and p-dimethylaminoazobenzene with microsomes isolated from adult guinea pigs maintained on a vitamin C free diet for only 12 days. These animals had no apparent signs of scurvy. In contrast to the earlier studies, these investigators showed that although the metabolism of aniline, hexobarbital, and zoxazolamine decreased, the metabolism of the other drugs was unchanged. They concluded that the effect of vitamin C deficiency was rather specific, particularly for hydroxylation reactions. Although many of the above studies established that ascorbic acid had an effect on drug metabolism, the underlying biochemical mechanism through which the vitamin was participating was unknown.

Our laboratory has been concerned with the role of the vitamin in the hepatic microsomal electron transport system (MFO); in determining if the vitamin affects subsequent detoxifying enzyme systems, such as epoxide hydrolase and glutathione transferase; in determining if the vitamin affects the binding of reactive intermediates such as epoxides to tissue macromolecules; and with its possible role in alcohol metabolism.

With regard to the hepatic microsomal MFO system, our studies with liver microsomes prepared from vitamin C deficient guinea pigs showed marked decreases in electron transport components such as cytochrome P-450 and NADPH cytochrome P-450 reductase. In addition, drug oxidative reactions such as aniline hydroxylation, aminopyrine N-demethylation, and p-nitroanisole O-demethylation were significantly decreased (Table 2-1) (15). A correlation between the concentrations of liver ascorbic acid and the quantity of cytochrome P-450 was also found in groups of guinea pigs on varying intakes of ascorbic acid (Figure 2-2) (16). The group with the highest quantity of cytochrome P-450 (24 nmol/100 mg of liver supernatant protein) had 2.5 times more of the heme protein than the ascorbic acid deficient group (9.6 nmol).

In vivo studies to determine the specificity of ascorbic acid indicated that other reducing agents, such as reduced 2,6-dichlorophenolindophenol (a dye with a similar redox potential to ascorbic acid), reduced glutathione, and D-isoascorbic acid, were not as effective as the vitamin in maintaining overall drug metabolism or the quantity of cytochrome P-450. For example, reduced glutathione did not significantly alter the liver microsomal cytochrome P-450 concentration, or p-nitroanisole O-demethylase activity. Ascorbyl palmitate, a more lipophilic form of the vitamin, however, was effective. The concentration of cytochrome P-450 was as high as found in the group of animals on a normal diet (17).

Kinetic studies to determine the apparent Michaelis-Menten affinity constant of a typical drug oxidation system, such as aminopyrine N-demethylation, indicated no difference in the apparent affinity constant in guinea pig microsomes prepared from deficient animals. In addition, there was no difference in the affinity constant in animals on a high intake of the vitamin (deficient, 1.67×10^{-3} M; normal diet, 1.67×10^{-3} M; normal diet plus 50 mg ascorbic acid per day, 1.57×10^{-3} M). Similar results were obtained in studies with O-demethylation of p-nitroanisole (6). In contrast to no difference in the apparent affinity

Table 2.1   Effect of Vitamin C Deficiency (21 days) on Electron Transport Components and Drug Enzymes in Guinea Pig Liver Microsomes[a]

	Activity		
	Normal	Vitamin C Deficient (21 days)	Decrease (%)
Cytochrome P-450[b]	0.05 ± 0.01	0.03 ± 0.003 $p < 0.01$	40
NADPH cytochrome[c] P-450 reductase	0.80 ± 0.2	< 0.01	85
Aniline hydroxylase[d]	1.6 ± 0.2	0.8 + 0.2 $p < 0.001$	50
Aminopyrine N-demethylase [d]	3.9 ± 0.1	1.7 ± 0.3 < 0.001	56
p-Nitroanisole[d] O-demethylase	3.2 ± 0.4	1.1 ± 0.2 < 0.001	66
Liver ascorbic acid Supernatant fraction 15,000 × g (μg/g wet weight)	194 ± 29	25 ± 15	
Microsomal fraction (μg/wet weight)	11 ± 3.8	3.5 ± 2.0	

[a]Mean ± SEM of 10 animals per group. Data from Zannoni, Flynn, and Lynch (15).
[b]Specific content equals μmoles/100 mg microsomal protein.
[c]Specific activity equals μmoles reduced/hr/100 mg of microsomal protein at 27°C.
[d]Specific activity equals μmoles of product formed/hr/100 mg of microsomal protein at 27°C.

for overall drug oxidation, there was a consistent alteration in the substrate, Type II-aniline-cytochrome P-450 binding spectrum in vitamin C deficient guinea pig microsomes. The binding spectrum was atypical in that the trough of the spectrum appeared at 405 nm instead of 390 nm, and the peak occurred at 440 nm instead of 430 nm. A marked decrease in absorption intensity was also observed at these wavelengths (15). In vitro experiments in which ascorbic acid was added to vitamin C deficient liver microsomes did not restore drug oxidation activities or NADPH cytochrome P-450 reductase activity, or alter the aniline-cytochrome P-450 binding spectrum. However, ascorbyl palmitate (2.3 × 10⁻³ M), the more lipophilic analog of ascorbic acid, did restore the atypical aniline-cytochrome P-450 binding spectra to its usual spectrum. The absorption intensity, however, was still significantly lower as were drug oxidation activities, which reflected the lower quantity of cytochrome P-450 in deficiency which could not be restored by the in vitro administration of either ascorbic acid or ascorbyl palmitate.

Reversal of decreased drug metabolism activities in vitamin C deficient animals by the in vitvo administration of ascorbic acid indicated that even though the concentration of liver ascorbic acid was restored to normal levels within 3 days, drug enzyme activities such as N-demethylation, O-demethylation, cytochrome P-450, and P-450 reductase required from 6 to 10 days of vitamin administration to return to normal. In addition, induction studies with phenobarbital indicated that overall

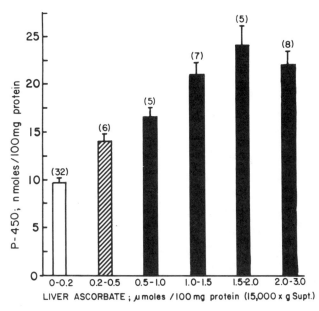

Figure 2-2. Correlation of hepatic cytochrome P-450 and ascorbic acid concentration. Cytochrome P-450 and ascorbic acid were determined in the liver 15,000 × g supernatant fraction from guinea pigs (200–250 g) maintained on an ascorbic acid deficient diet for 20 days (open bar), normal chow diet (cross-hatched bar) or chow diet plus 1.0 mg of ascorbic acid in the drinking water, daily (solid bars). Animals were divided into groups according to their liver concentration of ascorbic acid. One micromole of ascorbic acid per 100 mg of protein equals 19 mg/100 g wet weight of liver. Number in parentheses represents number of animals. Data from Rikans, Smith, and Zannoni (16).

drug oxidation activities, such as aniline hydroxylation, aminopyrine
N-demethylation, *p*-nitroanisole *O*-demethylation, and microsomal electron transport components, could be induced in vitamin C deficient
guinea pigs; the magnitude of induction was the same as found in normal animals (15).

The question was proposed whether ascorbic acid through its
antioxidant property could protect drug enzyme activities by inhibiting
lipid peroxidation; lipid peroxidation is known to be detrimental to the
MFO system. It was found, however, that lipid peroxidation was on the
order of 30% higher in microsomes isolated from normal guinea pigs
compared with microsomes isolated from guinea pigs on the ascorbic
acid deficient diet for 15 days (18). Although the quantity of the
phosphatidylcholine was slightly lower in the 15-day ascorbic acid deficient group compared with the normal group (18%), this decrease is
most likely not sufficient to immpair drug metabolism since 3-day-
starved guinea pigs fed ascorbic acid, which have increased drug metabolism activities (15), have a greater decrease in the quantity of
phosphatidylcholine than the 15-day ascorbic acid deficient group (19.2
μmol per 100 mg of microsomal protein compared to 22.4).

A determination of the concentration of liver ascorbic acid and
cytochrome P-450 indicated a relatively consistent quantitative relationship of ascorbic acid to cytochrome P-450. The ratio of liver ascorbic
acid to cytochrome P-450 was 2.2 in the ascorbic acid deficient group
and 2.3 in the normal group. When cytochrome P-450 was partially
purified from normal and ascorbic acid deficient guinea pig livers using
ammonium sulfate fractionation and calcium phosphate gel adsorption
and elution, the vitamin remained with cytochrome P-450 throughout
the fractionation procedure (18). The correlation between the concentration of liver ascorbic acid and cytochrome P-450 in microsomes prepared from normal and ascorbic acid deficient guinea pigs with partial
purification of cytochrome P-450 suggests that ascorbic acid may be directly associated with the heme protein. Metal chelators were employed
to investigate the possibility of ascorbic acid's involvement with the reduced form of iron of cytochrome P-450; that is, ferrous iron. It was
found that $\alpha,\acute{\alpha}$-dipyridyl, inhibited the formation of the CO binding
spectra of cytochrome P-450. The cytochrome P-450-CO binding decreased on the order of 50% in the presence of this chelator and could
be prevented by ascorbic acid. *o*-phenanthroline, another inhibitor with

a high affinity for ferrous iron, also inhibited the cytochrome P-450-CO binding spectrum which was also prevented by the vitamin.

Of the chelators tested, only ferrous iron chelators, such as $\alpha,\acute{\alpha}$-dipyridyl and o-phenanthroline significantly inhibited the cytochrome P-450-CO spectra (55% inhibition), while chelators with high affinity for copper, such as 8-diethyldithiocarbamate sulfonate bathocuproine, and diethyldithiocarbamate, were not significantly inhibitory (less than 5%). The apparent affinity constants of $\alpha,\acute{\alpha}$-dipyridyl for cytochrome P-450 are 2.99×10^{-4} M for normal and 3.14×10^{-4} M for ascorbic acid deficient microsomes. The apparent affinity constants for protection by ascorbic acid are 4.98×10^{-4} M for normal and 4.83×10^{-4} M for ascorbic acid deficient microsomes (18).

It was reported (8) that the administration of a precursor of heme, d-aminolevulinic acid (ALA), to vitamin C deficient guinea pigs caused an increase in the quantity of cytochrome P-450 (19). These findings suggested that ascorbic acid may be involved in the formation of heme. In view of this, it was important to determine if vitamin C deficiency affected the activity of ALA synthetase, the rate-limiting enzyme in heme synthesis, as well as other enzymes involved in heme synthesis, such as ALA dehydratase and ferrochelatase (Figure 2-3). As can be seen in Table 2-2, although cytochrome P-450 is markedly reduced in vitamin C

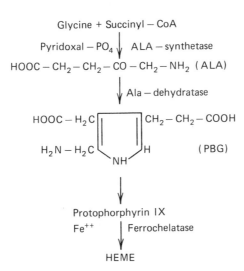

Figure 2-3. Pathway for the synthesis of heme from glycine and succinyl-CoA.

Table 2.2 Cytochrome P-450 and Heme Synthesis in Normal and Ascorbic Acid Deficient Guinea Pigs[a]

	Normal[b]	Deficient[c]
Cytochrome P-450[d] (nmol/100 mg protein)	19.2 ± 1.1	9.5 ± 0.7
ALA Synthetase (nmol ALA/hr/100 mg)	16.5 ± 2.3	18.1 ± 1.9
ALA Dehydratase (nmol PBG/hr/100 mg)	1056 ± 53	922 ± 33
Ferrochelatase (nmol ^{59}Fe/hr/100mg)	536 ± 33	589 ± 58

[a]Data from Rikans, Smith, and Zannoni (20).
[b]Normal guinea pigs; 1 mg ascorbic acid/mL in drinking water, daily. Liver ascorbic acid was 1740 nmoles/100 mg protein.
[c]Ascorbic acid deficient guinea pigs; on the diet for 20 days. Liver ascorbic acid was 99 nmoles/100 mg protein.
[d]Determined in liver 15,000 × g supernatant fraction.

deficient microsomes, there is no significant decrease in any of the key enzymes involved in heme synthesis. Similar results have recently been obtained by Walsch and Degkwitz (21). In addition, Omaye and Turnbull have reported that the decrease in cytochrome P-450 in ascorbic acid deficiency is not due to increased heme catabolism at least by way of induction of microsomal heme oxygenase activity (22).

An effect of ascorbic acid deficiency on different apo-forms of cytochrome P-450 was investigated in view of the finding of substantial depletion of the heme protein (15,18,23,24). It is well known that multiple forms of cytochrome P-450 exist in rabbit, rat, and mouse microsomes (25–32). These forms can be separated by gel electrophoresis in the presence of SDS. Our studies indicated that microsomes from guinea pigs indeed contain multiple forms of cytochrome P-450 in the 40,000 to 60,000 dalton region. Induction with phenobarbital and 3-methylcholanthrene and purification of the cytochromes indicate that a number of the guinea pig polypeptide bands with molecular weights from 44,000 to 60,000 contain cytochrome P-450, and the relative staining intensities of the bands reflect the quantity of different forms of cytochrome P-450. Microsomes from ascorbic acid deficient guinea pigs consistently demonstrated decreases in three of the polypeptide bands (molecular weights 44,000, 52,000, and 57,000) (Figure 2-4). Importantly, these differences were maintained in partially purified fractions from normal and ascorbic acid deficient guinea pigs (16). These results are in keeping with a selective action of ascorbic acid on specific forms of P-450 apoproteins. This selectivity is consistent with the effect of ascorbic acid deficiency in that the heme protein never decreased below 40 to 60% of normal even in a severely deficient state. Furthermore, that ascorbic acid deficiency may selectively affect certain forms of cytochrome P-450 is in keeping with the findings of Kuenzig and co-workers (24), who found that benzo(a)pyrene hydroxylase activity was unaltered in livers from deficient guinea pigs whereas 7-ethoxycoumarin dealkylase activity was less than 50% of normal.

We have recently found that ascorbic acid deficiency can also markedly affect particular MFO pathways of such environmental chemicals as bromobenzene and biphenyl. These compounds are interesting in that each of them is metabolized to intermediates requiring different forms of cytochrome P-450 (32,33). Bromobenzene is metabolized to *o*-bromophenol via 2,3-epoxidation and to *p*-bromophenol via 3,4-epoxidation (Figure 2-5). Biphenyl is metabolized either to a 2-hydroxylated product or to a 4-hydroxylated product. As can be seen in Table 2-3 the *p*-bromophenol pathway of bromobenzene and the 4-hydroxy pathway of biphenyl are significantly decreased in ascorbic acid deficiency, whereas the *o*-bromophenol and 2-hydroxylated biphenyl pathways are not statistically altered. These data are also in keeping with the finding and evidence for multiple forms of cytochrome

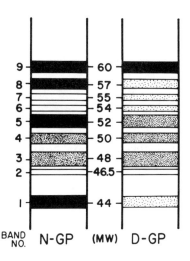

Figure 2-4. Schematic representation of SDS electrophoresis of liver microsomes prepared from normal and ascorbic acid deficient guinea pigs. Data from Rikans, Smith, and Zannoni (16).

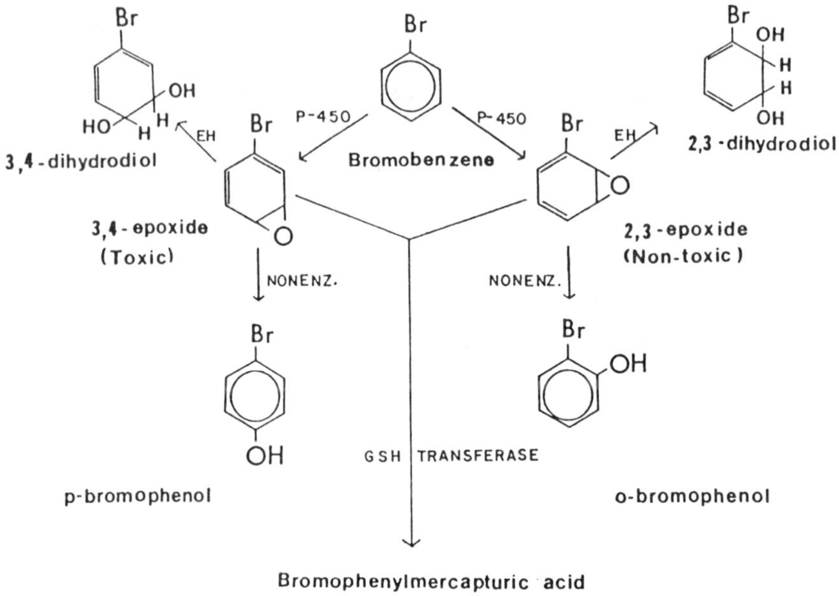

Figure 2-5.   Scheme of bromobenzene epoxidation via cytochrome P-450 mixed function oxidase system.

P-450, some of which are depleted in ascorbic acid deficiency whereas others are not affected.

It should be pointed out that a consequence of the metabolism of bromobenzene via the MFO system is the formation of reactive 2,3- and 3,4-epoxide intermediates. The 3,4-epoxide metabolite of bromobenzene is particularly detrimental in that it leads to severe hepatic centrilobular necrosis by covalent binding to tissue proteins (34). In a search for agents which could protect against such tissue damage we found that the lipophilic analog of ascorbic acid, ascorbyl palmitate, was very effective in blocking adduct formation (35). It was, in fact, as effective as known protective agents such as glutathione or cysteine (Table 2-4). The significance and importance of the protective role of this lipophilic analog of ascorbic acid with bromobenzene or other environmental chemicals which bind covalently to tissue macromolecules or, for that matter, DNA warrant further investigation.

The mammalian cell has other important mechanisms to protect against the detrimental effects of electrophilic metabolites which may

Table 2.3 Bromobenzene and Biphenyl Hydroxylation via the Hepatic MFO System in Normal and Ascorbate Deficient Guinea Pig[a]

Guinea pigs[b]	P-450[c]	Bromobenzene[d]		Biphenyl[d]	
		o-BP	p-BP	2-OH	4-OH
Normal (15)	0.19 ± .01	9.3 ± 0.9	122 ± 8	22 ± 1.0	164 ± 8
Deficient (11)	0.07 ± .01	6.3 ± 0.5	53 ± 9	19 ± 2.0	86 ± 2

[a]Data from Zannoni, Holsztynska, and Lau (33). Mean ± SEM given; number in parentheses equals number of animals.
[b]Number in parenthesis equals number of animals.
[c]nmoles/mg of 15,000 × g supernatant protein.
[d]nmoles product/min/100 mg microsomal protein.
[e]Difference not significant.
[f]Significant difference from normal $p < 0.01$.

Table 2.4 Effect of Various Agents on the Covalent Binding of 3,4- and 2,3-Bromobenzene Oxides to Rat Liver Microsomal Protein[a]

Additions (1.0 mM)	Phenobarbital Induced Microsomes[b]		3-Methylcholanthrene Induced Microsomes[c]	
	Specific Binding nmole/min/100 mg Microsomal Protein	Inhibition (%)	Specific Binding nmole/min/100 mg Microsomal Protein	Inhibition (%)
None	94 + 2 (5)	0	75 ± 2 (4)	0
Ascorbyl palmitate	32[d] ± 2 (4)	68	32[d] ± 1 (4)	57
Glutathione	34[d] ± 2 (4)	65	31[d] ± 2 (4)	59
Cysteine	47[d] ± 3 (4)	51	24[d] ± 2 (4)	68
Ascorbic acid	86 ± 2 (4)	9	64 ± 3 (4)	15
Palmitic acid	89 ± 2 (3)	5	92 ± 5 (3)	−23
Vitamin E	107 ± 4 (3)	−14	63 ± 4 (3)	16

[a]Number in parentheses equals the number of individual experiments; mean ± SEM. Data modified from Zannoi, Marker, and Lau (35).
[b]The epoxidation of bromobenzene (3.0 mM) to p-bromophenol via its 3,4- oxide was enhanced by pretreating rats with phenobarbital.
[c]The epoxidation of bromobezene (3.0 mM) to o-bromophenol via its 2,3- oxide was enhances by pretreating rats with 3-methylcholanthrene.
[d]$p < 0.001$ with respect to control.

lead to necrosis or carcinogenesis. These detoxification mechanisms involve enzymatic reactions utilizing glutathione or water; glutathione transferase and epoxide hydrolase are such enzyme systems (Figure 2-6). It was of interest to determine if either hydrolase or transferase was affected by ascorbic acid deficiency. As indicated in Table 2-5 there is no significant difference in either the specific activity or the apparent affinity of hepatic epoxide hydrolase for styrene oxide in microsomes isolated from ascorbic acid deficient or normal guinea pigs. Furthermore, groups of animals on high intake of ascorbic acid showed no difference in epoxide hydrolase activity when compared to deficient animals or animals on a normal intake of the vitamin. The animals in this study were pair-fed. Animals on a normal Purina chow diet, however, showed on the order of a 35% increase in hydrolase activity compared to groups of animals on a Nutritional Biochemical ascorbic acid deficient diet. The Purina normal diet contained 2.25 parts per million of the antioxidant food additive BHA, which appears to be responsible for the increase in hydrolase activity. We have shown this increase with groups of animals on a diet with 5 parts per million BHA. This food additive is a known

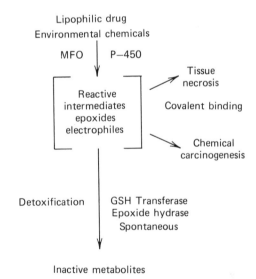

Figure 2-6. Pathways for the metabolism and detoxification of drugs and environmental chemicals via the mixed function oxygenase, glutathione transferase, and epoxide hydrase pathway.

Table 2.5   Hepatic Epoxide Hydrolase and Glutathione Transferase in Normal and Ascorbic Acid Deficient Guinea Pigs[a]

		Hydrolase Activity[b]	K_m	GSH Transferase Activity[c] Activity[c]
Normal	(A)	52.2 ± 6 (3)	465 μM	421
	(B)	45.7 ± 3 (6)		
Deficient		50.0 ± 5 (4)	398 μM	416

[a]Unpublished data; R. C. Smart and V. G. Zannoni. Guinea pigs (Hartley) male, 215–225 g; groups were pair-fed for 19 days with ascorbate deficient diet. Normal (A) group was supplemented with 1.0 mg ascorbate/mL drinking water daily, liver ascorbate, 21 mg/100 g. Normal (B) group was supplemented with 2.0 mg ascorbate/mL drinking water daily, liver ascorbate, 38 mg/100 g. Deficient diet group; liver ascorbate, 2.5 mg/100 g. Number in parentheses equals number of experiments, ±SD.
[b]nmoles of product/min/mg washed microsomes at 37°C; substrate styrene oxide with tetrahydrofuran.
[c]nmoles of product min/mg of 100,000 × g supernatant at 27°C, substrate p-NO$_2$ benzylchloride.

inducer of mouse and rat epoxide hydrolase (36). As was found with epoxide hydrolase, glutathione transferase activity (33) was also not significantly altered in vitamin C deficiency (Table 2-5). With regard to the participation of ascorbic acid in alleviating the consequences of reactive metabolites, it should be emphasized that the effect of the vitamin would rely heavily on the particular form of cytochrome P-450 jeopardized. Also of importance is the vitamin's availability to chemically protect, via its reducing properties, against adduct formation and not its influence on the latter stages of detoxification involving hydrolase or transferase.

With respect to the involvement of ascorbic acid with cytochrome P-450, it has been of recent interest that this heme protein is involved in ethanol metabolism (37). In studies to determine if the microsomal ethanol oxidizing system (MEOS) was compromised in ascorbic acid deficiency, we found no significant difference in the specific activity of MEOS in ascorbic acid deficient microsomes from those isolated from normal guinea pigs. However, there was a marked effect of ascorbic acid incubated with 100,000 × g hepatic supernatant or mitochondrial fractions in that ethanol was metabolized to acetaldehyde and methanol was metabolized to formaldehyde in the presence of the vitamin (Table 2-6).

Table 2.6   The In Vitro Effect of Ascorbic Acid on the Oxidation of Methanol and Ethanol[a]

Guinea Pig Liver Preparation	Activity (nmoles/min/mg of protein at 37°C)	
	Substrate	Substrate
	Methanol[b]	Ethanol[c]
100,000 × g fraction	187	176
Mitochondrial fraction	160	170
Microsomal fraction	nd	nd

[a]Unpublished data; R. L. Susick and V. G. Zannoni. nd = not detectable.
[b]The metabolism of methanol was determined by incubating the liver fraction (12 μg of protein) with 200 μmoles of substrate and 2 μmoles of ascorbic acid in sodium phosphate buffer (0.1M, pH 6.8) containing 10 μmoles of o-phenathroline. The total volume was 1.0 mL; formaldehyde was measured according to the method of Nash (38).
[c]The metabolism of ethanol was determined as described for methanol except 200 μmoles of ethanol was used as the substrate. Acetaldehyde was measured by gas chromatography according to the method of Ohnishi (39).

The importance of ascorbic acid in the catalysis of methanol or ethanol via perhaps the known systems, such as alcohol dehydrogenase or catalase, or for that matter via a heretofore unknown enzymatic or nonenzymatic route, is in need of further investigation.

REFERENCES

1.   A. H. Conney and J. J. Burns, *Adv. Pharmacol.,* **1**, 31 (1962).

2.   A. H. Conney, *Pharmacol. Rev.,* **19**, 317 (1967).

3.   A. H. Conney, *Fundamentals of Drug Metabolism and Drug Disposition* (B. N. La Du, H. G. Mandel, and E. L. Way, Eds.), Baltimore, Williams and Wilkins, 1971, 13, 253.

4.   V. G. Zannoni and P. H. Sato, *Fed. Proc.,* **33**, 546 (1976).

5.   V. G. Zannoni and M. M. Lynch, *Drug Metab. Rev.,* **2**, 57 (1973).

6.   V. G. Zannoni and P. H. Sato, *Ann. N.Y. Acad. Sci.,* **258**, 119 (1975).

7.   E. Ginter, *Ann. N.Y. Acad. Sci.,* **258**, 410 (1975).

8.   E. Degkwitz and H. Staundinger, *Hoppe-Seyler's Z. Physiol. Chem.,* **342**, 63 (1965).

9.   E. Degkwitz, P. Luft, U. Pfeiffer, and H. Staundinger, *Hoppe-Seyler's Z. Physiol. Chem.,* **349**, 465 (1968).

10. R. K. Richards, K. Jueter, and T. I. Klatt, *Proc. Soc. Exper. Biol. Med.*, **48,** 403 (1941).

11. J. Axelrod, S. Udenfriend, and B. B. Brodie, *J. Pharmacol. Exp. Therap.*, **111,** 176 (1954).

12. A. H. Conney, G. A. Bray, C. Evans, and J. J. Burns, *Ann. N.Y. Acad. Sci.*, **92,** 115 (1961).

13. H. Leber, E. Degkwitz, and H. Staundinger, *Hoppe-Seyler's Z. Physiol. Chem.*, **350,** 439 (1969).

14. R. Kato, A. Takanaka, and T. Oshima, *Japan. J. Pharmacol.*, **19,** 25 (1969).

15. V. G. Zannoni, E. J. Flynn, and M. M. Lynch, *Biochem. Pharmacol.*, **21,** 1377 (1972).

16. L. E. Rikans, C. R. Smith, and V. G. Zannoni, *J. Pharmacol. Exp. Therap.*, **204,** 702 (1978).

17. P. H. Sato and V. G. Zannoni, *Biochem. Pharm.*, **23,** 312 (1974).

18. P. H. Sato and V. G. Zannoni, *J. Pharmacol. Exp. Therap.*, **198,** 295 (1976).

19. D. Luft, L. Degkwitz, Hochli-Kaufmann, and H. Staundinger, *Hoppe-Seyler's Z. Physiol. Chem.*, **353,** 1420 (1972).

20. L. E. Rikans, C. R. Smith, and V. G. Zannoni, *Biochem. Pharmacol.*, **26,** 797 (1977).

21. S. Walsch and E. Degkwitz, *Hoppe-Seyler's Z. Physiol. Chem.*, **361,** 79 (1980).

22. S. T. Omaye and J. D. Turnbull, *Biochem. Pharmacol.*, **28,** 1415 (1979).

23. E. Degkwitz, S. Walsch, and M. Dubberstein, *Hoppe-Seyler's Z. Physiol. Chem.*, **355,** 1152 (1974).

24. W. Kuenzig, V. Tkaczevski, J. J. Kamm, A. H. Conney, and J. J. Burns, *J. Pharmacol. Exp. Therap.*, **201,** 527 (1977).

25. T. A. van der Hoeven and M. J. Coon, *J. Biol. Chem.*, **249,** 6302 (1974).

26. C. Hashimoto and Y. Imai, *Biochem. Biophys. Res. Commun.*, **68,** 821 (1976).

27. D. Ryan, A. Y. H. Lu, J. Kawalek, S. B. West, and W. Levin, *Biochem. Biophys. Res. Commun.*, **64,** 1134 (1975).

28. A. F. Welton and S. D. Aust, *Biochem. Biophys. Res. Commun.*, **56,** 898 (1974).

29. A. F. Welton, F. O'Neal, L. C. Chaney, and S. D. Aust, *J. Biol. Chem.*, **250,** 5631 (1975).

30. M. Huang, S. B. West, and A. Y. H. Lu, *J. Biol. Chem.*, **251,** 4659 (1976).

31. D. A. Haugen, T. A. van der Hoeven, and M. J. Coon, *J. Biol. Chem.*, **250,** 3567 (1975).

32. S. S. Lau and V. G. Zannoni, *Toxicol. Appl. Pharmacol.*, **50,** 309 (1979).

33. V. G. Zannoni, E. J. Holsztynska, and S. S. Lau, *Ascorbic Acid Chemistry, Metabolism and Uses, Advances in Chemistry Series*, P. A. Seib and P. M. Tolbert, Eds., Washington, D.C., American Chemical Society, 1982, pp. 349–368.

34. S. S. Lau, G. D. Abrams, and V. G. Zannoni, *J. Pharmacol. Exp. Therap.*, **214,** 703 (1980).

35. V. G. Zannoni, E. K. Marker, and S. S. Lau, *Drug-Nutrient Interactions*, **1,** 193 (1982).

36. Y. Cha, F. Martz, and E. Bueding, *Cancer Res.*, **38,** 4496 (1978).

37. C. S. Lieber and L. M. DeCarli, *J. Biol. Chem.*, **245,** 2505 (1970).

38. E. J. Flynn, M. Lynch, and V. G. Zannoni, *Biochem. Pharmacol.*, **21,** 2577 (1972).

39. K. Ohnishi and C. S. Lieber, *J. Biol. Chem.*, **252,** 7124 (1977).

3

Trace Metals in Human Nutrition

HAROLD H. SANDSTEAD, M.D.

USDA/ARS Human Nutrition Research Center, Grand Forks, North Dakota

The role of trace elements in human nutrition has, to a large extent, been clarified since 1950 (1). Whereas the importance of iodine, iron, fluorine, and cobalt for human nutrition was established in the first half of this century, requirements for other trace elements were only inferred from research on plants and animals. In fact, their wide distribution in the environment suggested to some reviewers that deficiencies were unlikely. Analysis of human tissues had revealed concentrations of trace elements that were similar to those in other higher animals. This, along with other chemical similarities, supported the notion that trace element functions in humans were similar to those in other animals. Because there was limited clinical evidence of deficiencies or other diseases related to abnormal trace element nutriture with the exception of the trace elements noted above, and because analytical techniques were laborious, clinical investigation of trace elements was, with few exceptions, limited to the elements noted above. Advances in technology that made atomic absorption spectroscopy widely available did much to change this situation. This technique and the more recently available plasma emission spectroscopy have made analysis of trace elements accessible to many investigators and practicing physicians. Thus interest in trace elements and their importance in human metabolism has been heightened. As a result of this increased awareness, deficiencies of nine of the 14–17 trace elements required or beneficial for animal species have been recognized in humans. The nine include iodine, iron, zinc, copper, chromium, selenium, molybdenum, manganese, and cobalt. In addition, cadmium and methylmercury have joined lead as toxic elements affecting the health of large numbers of people. Advances in knowledge of the role of trace elements in nutrition and metabolism of humans and other species are now coming with amazing rapidity. Trace elements such as nickel, arsenic, and boron, whose essentiality seemed very unlikely a few years ago, are now known to be required in parts per billion amounts by rats and chicks. One wonders about their importance in human nutrition and metabolism.

Comprehensive reviews of trace elements and their roles in metabolism are available (1–6). This chapter is limited to a few key discoveries and an important principle of trace element metabolism that seem particularly relevant to human health.

ZINC

One of the major trace element discoveries of the last 20 years was recognition of zinc deficiency among adolescents in Iran and Egypt by Prasad (7,8). Human zinc deficiency had previously been thought unlikely because of zinc's wide abundance in the environment; research had therefore focused primarily on other species. Prasad did not accept this notion; and through a series of studies, characterized the syndrome and changed the scientific landscape with regard to zinc. Prasad's patients displayed severe growth failure, delayed sexual maturation, and other endocrine findings similar to hypopituitarism. They were frequently iron deficient. Their zinc kinetics were consistent with the diagnosis of zinc deficiency and their responses to treatment with zinc and an otherwise adequate diet established the diagnosis. Subsequent work by many workers who studied various species revealed many biochemical and physiologic functions of zinc. Zinc is now known to be necessary for activity of more than 200 enzymes from various species and appears essential for genetic expression (9). Some examples of processes that require zinc include nucleic acid and protein synthesis; cell division and hypertrophy; tissue growth and maturation; cellular and humoral immunity; epithelial integrity and wound healing; sexual maturation and function; neuropsychological function; the special senses including vision, smell, and taste; appetite; and metabolism of carbon dioxide and superoxide (7,8). With such important roles in metabolism it is perhaps surprising that human deficiency of zinc was not recognized sooner. The delay in recognition was probably related to the difficulties associated with measurement of zinc prior to the advent of atomic absorption spectroscopy. Other factors may have been the geographic distribution of the syndrome, the preoccupation of human nutrition researchers in the third world with other deficiencies of major importance, including protein-energy malnutrition, iron deficiency, vitamin A deficiency, and folic acid deficiency, and the opinion of many researchers that trace element deficiencies were highly unlikely in humans.

It now appears that zinc deficiency related to diet occurs throughout the world (7,8). It is most common among poor populations that subsist primarily on cereals and other foods of vegetable origin. These foods are poor sources of bioavailable zinc because of their hemicellulose, lignin, and phytate contents (10). Cooking methods that result in formation of Maillard browning products, potent chelators of zinc, may also decrease zinc bioavailability. Because red meat, organ meats, and certain crustaceans and shellfish are the best dietary sources of zinc, populations that infrequently eat these foods have an increased risk of deficiency (11). Research utilizing U.S. diets that included a variety of foods has shown from balance studies that dietary phosphorus and protein are important determinants of zinc requirement (10). Regression analysis of data from balance studies indicates that requirement increases as dietary phosphorus and protein increase. Other studies have shown that inhibitors of zinc absorption included fractions of dietary fiber and that phytate and calcium interact to inhibit zinc absorption (12). It is from studies such as these that the importance of food type and food selection in the pathogenesis of zinc deficiency has been established.

Zinc deficiency in humans also occurs secondary to disease conditions. These include a genetic zinc malabsorption disorder, acrodermatitis enteropathica, the human analog of lethal trait A46 of cattle, and diseases that either impair absorption or increase excretion of zinc (7,8,10,13).

Available evidence suggests that zinc deficiency is a worldwide problem. Its true impact on human health and productivity is just beginning to be appreciated. As requirement is relatively increased at times of rapid growth, pregnant women, infants, children, and adolescents are at greatest risk of deficiency. Experimental findings in animals suggest that organ systems such as the brain, with a well defined period of rapid growth and maturation, are highly susceptible to injury from zinc deficiency and that sequelae from injury are persistent (7,14,15). These findings in animals are probably applicable to humans.

IRON

Inspired by the fact that iron deficiency is the most widespread nutritional deficiency in the world, researchers have characterized factors involved in its pathogenesis. Moore (16) and others established that iron is more available for absorption from meat than from foods of vegetable origin, and that ascorbic acid facilitates the absorption of iron from vegetables. Subsequently, Layrisse (17) and others showed the wide differences in iron bioavailability from cereals and legumes compared to meat. Substances in food that inhibit or facilitate iron absorption have been identified, as have pathologic conditions affecting iron nutriture. Extensive knowledge of factors that affect iron bioavailability has made it possible to evaluate diets for their adequacy as sources of iron (18,19).

Research on iron deficiency has focused to a large extent on diagnosis, effects of anemia, iron metabolism, and iron bioavailability. Recently, functional effects of deficient iron nutriture have received increased attention. Impairments in physical work performance (20), thyroid function, and temperature regulation (21) have been identified. Impairments in work capacity by iron deficiency anemia have been shown to have significant economic impacts on workers because of decreases in their productivity. This finding appears particularly important for third world countries, where iron deficiency is prevalent and income is primarily derived from physical labor. Studies in iron deficient rats have shown impaired temperature regulation in response to cold, and defective conversion of T_4 to T_3. Preliminary studies in humans have revealed similar relationships. Their significance, if any, for work performance remains to be identified.

Another finding that seems of potential importance in both the developed and undeveloped world is the discovery that central nervous system function is influenced by iron nutriture (22,23). Iron deficient preschool children were found to have deficits in attention and cognition that were responsive to iron therapy. The significance of these findings for school performance and subsequent productivity is speculative. At the very least, it seems likely that attention in school is compromised. In adults, recent research has shown correlations between iron nutriture, cognition, and electrophysiologic indices in persons who were not iron deficient by usual standards. Both EEG lateralization and power were related to iron stores, indexed by serum ferritin. Cognitive performance was correlated with iron stores, and related to the EEG. These findings suggest that neuropsychological function is far more sensitive to iron nutriture than has previously been appreciated. Clarification of the implication of these findings for daily living awaits further research.

COPPER

Another discovery, whose significance is still emerging, is that many U.S. diets contain substantially less copper than was previously believed (24). The amounts are in a range where maintenance of copper homeostasis may be difficult. Epidemiologic studies and observations on experimental animals suggest that habitually low intakes of dietary copper can adversely affect cardiovascular health (25). Recognition of the importance of copper nutriture for cardiovascular health has transformed copper from an esoteric nutrient to one of potential public health significance. Many dietary and physiologic factors that influence copper nutriture have been identified. It appears that dietary zinc, protein, fiber, and phytate influence copper bioavailability and thus dietary requirement. As dietary zinc, phytate, or fiber increases, copper retention is apparently impaired. Increasing dietary protein improves retention of copper, perhaps through facilitation of copper absorption by certain amino acids or peptides.

Copper deficiency in experimental animals causes many sequelae. Abnormalities that seem to have implications for human health include impairment of glucose metabolism (26), abnormal lipid metabolism and hypercholesterolemia (27), cardiac necrosis (28), dissecting aneurysm (29), osteopenia and fracture (30), impaired myelinization (31), anemia and leukopenia (30), and congenital anomalies (32). In humans, experimental copper deficiency has impaired glucose utilization (33) and elevated serum cholesterol (34). Osteopenia, fracture, anemia, and leukopenia have been described in copper deficient infants (30). Impaired myelinization and arterial aneurysms may be seen in infants with an inborn error of copper utilization known as Menkies' syndrome (35). Research in progress will show if any of these phenomena have relevance for the population at large.

CHROMIUM

Chromium is another trace element that has emerged as having an important role in human metabolism. Evidence of chromium responsive insulin resistance in humans (36) is consistent with findings in chromium deficient animals that chromium facilitates the action of insulin (37). The potential importance of chromium in human health was suggested many years ago by Schroeder (38). He reported that tissue chromium concentrations of North Americans tend to decrease with age, and speculated that the decrease was related in some way to consumption of highly refined diets. He noted that refining removed much of the chromium from foods. Based on his own research and that of Mertz (37), he speculated that impaired chromium nutriture among North Americans was a factor in the occurrence of diabetes mellitus and atherosclerotic cardiovascular disease.

Severe human chromium deficiency has been described in a patient who received chromium deficient total intravenous alimentation for many months (39). She displayed impaired glucose and amino acid utilization, poor responsiveness to exogenous insulin, weakness, weight loss, and peripheral neuropathy. Chromium supplementation corrected these problems.

Chromium supplementation has been given to patients as inorganic trivalent chromium, or as an organic complex as brewer's yeast. Brewer's yeast is a good source of "glucose tolerance factor," an as yet incompletely characterized organic chromium compound. Adults given brewer's yeast have shown improved glucose clearance and lower serum cholesterol (40). Other adults with adult onset diabetes have shown improved glucose metabolism when given inorganic trivalent chromium (41). These findings confirm the essentiality of chromium for humans. Their significance for the population at large awaits further research.

SELENIUM

Selenium is an element whose deficiency and toxicity are of unquestioned importance in animal husbandry (1). Until recently, however, it seemed very unlikely that selinium deficiency was more than a very rare problem in humans. Discovery in China that cardiomyopathy and death among children from Keshan Province was caused by selenium deficiency, possibly complicated by a virus infection, showed that humans as well as farm animals who live on foods raised on selenium deficient soil are at risk of selenium deficiency (42). Grains raised in the region were low in selenium, as was blood from persons living on farms where selenium deficiency occurred in farm animals. Selenium supplementation of the populace nearly eliminated the occurrence of the cardiomyopathy. Subsequent studies in mice showed that selenium deficiency predisposed the mice to cardiomyopathy and death when they were given a Coxsackie B4 virus that had been isolated from a child who died of Keshan disease. These findings from China demonstrate that humans who consume foods from a limited geographic area have a potential risk of deficiencies or toxicities of essential or toxic elements, similar to farm animals.

LEAD

The insidious nature of lead poisoning in humans is exemplified by evidence of abnormal neuropsychological sequelae in school children who were apparently exposed to increased environmental lead several years previously (43,44). Evidence of earlier exposure was elevated lead in deciduous teeth or hair. Neuropsychological sequelae included attentional deficits and a small decrement in IQ. While the significance of these effects for daily living is unclear, it is probable they are not beneficial. These findings in school children have been somewhat controversial, apparently because of disagreements about methodology (45). Other evidence suggests that the lead burden of many U.S. children is greater than previously suspected. Blood lead concentrations of children who participated in the second National Health and Nutrition Examination Survey revealed a surprisingly high incidence of elevated levels among children from the central part of large cities, and black children (46). These discoveries should alert us of the need for careful monitoring of environmental toxins such as lead, cadmium, and mercury for evaluation of their functional effects on segments of the population that are at greatest risk of injury (pregnant and lactating women, infants, and children).

METAL INTERACTIONS

A fundamental concept in trace element research that has facilitated understanding of their roles in biology, and their relations one to another, is the idea that elements that are chemically similar behave similarly in biological systems (47). Their similarity causes them to compete for biological ligands. A clinically important example of this phenomenon is the competition between zinc and copper for intestinal absorption (24). This interaction probably accounts for the recently discovered beneficial effects of oral zinc supplements on patients with hepatolenticular degeneration (Wilson's disease) (48), and provides a basis for the suggestion that intakes of zinc that exceed nutritional needs can be harmful. An experiment showing toxicity of oral zinc supplements was reported in young men (49). They were given 160 mg zinc by mouth daily. The principal manifestation of toxicity was a decline in plasma HDL-cholesterol. The mechanism of the effect appears to have been an inhibition of intestinal absorption of copper (24). Impaired copper nutriture is known to adversely affect lipid and cholesterol metabolism. Examples of other interactions that appear important for human health are those between the toxic elements, cadmium, lead, and methylmercury, and certain essential elements (50). Research in animals has led to the suggestion that dietary iron, zinc, copper, and selenium may help protect humans from intoxication by environmental levels of these elements (51).

REFERENCES

1. E. J. Underwood, Ed., *Trace Elements in Human and Animal Nutrition*, New York, Academic, 1976.

2. A. S. Prasad, Ed., *Trace Elements in Human Health and Disease*, Vols. I and II, New York, Academic, 1976.

3. F. Bronner and J. W. Coburn, Eds., *Disorders of Mineral Metabolism, Vol. I, Trace Minerals*, New York, Academic, 1981.

4. A. S. Prasad, Ed., *Clinical, Biochemical, and Nutritional Aspects of Trace Elements*, New York, Alan R. Liss, 1982.

5. B. Sarkar, Ed., *Biological Aspects of Metals and Metal-Related Diseases*, New York, Raven, 1983.

6. I. E. Dreosti and R. M. Smith, Eds., *Neurobiology of the Trace Elements*, Volume I, New Jersey, Humana, 1983.

7. H. H. Sandstead, in F. Bronner and J. W. Coburn, Eds., *Disorders of Mineral Metabolism*, Vol. I, *Trace Minerals*, New York, Academic, 1981, pp. 93–157.

8. A. S. Prasad, in *Clinical, Biochemical, and Nutritional Aspects of Trace Elements*, New York, Alan R. Liss, 1982, pp. 3–62.

9. B. L. Vallee and K. H. Falchuk, in B. Sarkar, Ed., *Biological Aspects of Metals and Metal-Related Diseases*, New York, Raven, 1983, pp. 1–14.

10. H. H. Sandstead, in A. S. Prasad, Ed., *Clinical, Biochemical, and Nutritional Aspects of Trace Elements*, New York, Alan R. Liss, 1982, pp. 83–101.

11.   H. H. Sandstead, L. K. Henriksen, J. L. Greger, A. S. Prasad, and R. A. Good, *Am. J. Clin. Nutr.,* **36,** 1046 (1982).

12.   H. H. Sandstead, Bioavailability of Zinc for Intestinal Absorption from Human Diets, Symposium at Maharry College in Nashville, in press, *Am. J. Clin. Nutr.,* 1984.

13.   H. H. Sandstead, K. P . Vo-Khactu, and N. Solomons, in A. S. Prasad, Ed., *Trace Elements in Human Health and Disease,* Vol. I, New York, Academic, 1976, pp. 181–187.

14.   H. H. Sandstead, J. C. Wallwork, E. S. Halas, D. M. Tucker, C. L. Dverstedn, and D. A. Strobel, in B. Sarkar, Ed., *Biological Aspects of Metals and Metal-Related Diseases,* New York, Raven, 1983, pp. 225–241.

15.   E. S. Halas, in I. E. Dreosti and R. M. Smith, Eds., *Neurobiology of the Trace Elements,* Volume I, New Jersey, Humana, 1983, pp. 213–243.

16.   C. V. Moore, in R. S. Goodhart and M. Shils, Eds., *Modern Nutrition in Health and Disease,* Philadelphia, Lea & Febiger, 1973, pp. 297–323.

17.   M. Layrisse and C. M. Torres, *Progress in Hematology,* Vol. VII, 137, (1971).

18.   E. R. Monsen, L. Halberg, M. Layrisse, D. M. Hegsted, J. D. Cook, W. Mertz, and C. A. Finch, *Am. J. Clin. Nutr.,* **31,** 134 (1978).

19.   Iron, in Recommended Dietary Allowances, 9th Edition, National Academy Science/National Research Council, Washington, D. C., 1980, pp. 137–144.

20.   V. R. Edgerton, Y. Ohira, G. W. Gardner, and B. Senewiratne, in E. Pollitt and R. L. Leibel, Eds., *Iron Deficiency: Brain Biochemistry and Behavior,* New York, Raven, 1982, pp. 141–160.

21.   E. Dillman, B. Mackler, D. Johnson, G. Brengelmann, W. Green, C. Gale, J. Martin, M. Layrisse, C. Martinez-Torres, and C. Finch, in E. Pollit and R. L. Leibel, Eds., *Iron Deficiency: Brain Biochemistry and Behavior,* New York, Raven, 1982, pp. 57–62.

22.   E. Pollitt, F. Viteri, C. Saco-Pollitt, and R. L. Leibel, in E. Pollitt and R. L. Leibel, Eds., *Iron Deficiency: Brain Biochemistry and Behavior,* New York, Raven, 1982, pp. 195–208.

23.   D. M. Tucker, H. H. Sandstead, J. G. Penland, S. R. Dawson, and D. B. Milne, Iron status and brain function: serum ferritin levels associated with asymmetries of cortical electrophysiology and cognitive performance. *Am. J. Clin. Nutr.,* 1984 (in press).

24.   H. H. Sandstead, *Am. J. Clin. Nutr.,* **35,** 809 (1982).

25.   L. M. Klevay, *Ann. N. Y. Acad. Sci.,* **355,** 140 (1980).

26.   M. Fields, R. J. Ferrette, J. C. Smith, and S. Reiser, *J. Nutr.,* **113,** 1335 (1983).

27.   K. G. D. Allen and L. M. Klevay, *Atherosclerosis,* **31,** 259 (1978).

28.   K. G. D. Allen and L. M. Klevay, *Atherosclerosis,* **29,** 81 (1978).

29.   B. L. O'Dell, R. B. Hardwick, G. Reynolds, and J. E. Savage, *Proc. Soc. Exp. Biol. and Med.,* **108,** 402 (1961).

30.   A. Cordano, J. M. Baertl, and G. G. Graham, *Pediatrics,* 324 (1964).

31.   W. W. Carlton and W. A. Kelley, *J. Nutr.,* **97,** 42 (1969).

32.   L. S. Hurley, *Physio. Rev.,* **61,** 249 (1981).

33.   L. M. Klevay, W. K. Canfield, S. K. Gallagher, L. K. Henriksen, W. Bolunchuk, L. K. Johnson, H. C. Lukaski, D. B. Milne, and H. H. Sandstead. *Clin. Res.,* **30,** 780A (1982); *AJCN,* **37,** 717 (1983); *Clin. Res.,* **31,** 618A (1983).

34.   L. M. Klevay, L. Inman, L. K. Johnson, M. R. Lawler, J. R. Mahalko, D. B. Milne, and H. H. Sandstead, *Clin. Res.,* **28,** 758A (1980).

35. D. M. Danks, P. E. Campbell, B. J. Stevens, V. Mayne, and E. Cartwright, *Pediatrics,* **50,** 188 (1972).

36. R. Riales and M. J. Albrink, *Am. J. Clin. Nutr.,* **34,** 2670 (1981).

37. W. Mertz, *Physiol. Rev.,* **49,** 163 (1969).

38. H. A. Schroeder, A. P. Nason, and I. H. Tipton, *J. Chronic Dis.,* **23,** 123 (1970).

39. K. N. Jeejeebhoy, R. Chi, E. B. Marliss, G. R. Greenbey, and A. Bruce-Robertson, *Am. J. Clin. Nutr.,* **30,** 531 (1977).

40. E. G. Offenbacker and F. X. Pi-Sunyer, *Diabetes,* **29,** 919 (1980).

41. R. A. Levine, D. H. P. Streeten, and R. J. Doisy, *Metabolism,* **17,** 114 (1968).

42. K. Ge, in M. Winick, Ed., *Adolescent Nutrition,* New York, Wiley, 1982, pp. 127–138.

43. H. L. Needleman, *New Eng. J. Med.,* **300,** 689 (1979).

44. R. W. Thatcher, M. L. Lester, R. McAlaster, and R. Horst, *Arch. Env. Health,* **37,** 159 (1982).

45. E. Marshall, *Science,* **222,** 906 (1983).

46. K. R. Mahaffee, J. L. Annest, J. Roberts, and R. S. Murphy, *New Eng. J. Med.,* **307,** 573 (1982).

47. C. H. Hill and G. Matrone, *Fed. Proc.,* **29,** 1474 (1970).

48. G. J. Brewer, G. M. Hill, A. S. Prasad, Z. T. Cossack, and P. Rabbani, *Ann. Int. Med.,* **99,** 314 (1983).

49. P. L. Hooper, L. Visconti, P. J. Garry, and G. E. Johnson, *JAMA,* **244,** 17, 1960 (1980).

50. H. H. Sandstead, *J. Lab. Clin. Med.,* **98,** 457 (1981).

51. M. R. S. Fox, *J. Food Science,* **39,** 321 (1974).

4

Nutrition During Pregnancy: Myths and Realities

P. ROSSO, M.D.

Institute of Human Nutrition, Columbia University College of Physicians and Surgeons, New York, New York

The importance of maternal nutrition during pregnancy has been the subject of much controversy. Although there seems to be general agreement that severe undernutrition reduces mean birth weight, the relevance of nutrition for women living in Western industrialized countries is disputed. The issue revolves around the problem of whether an everyday diet influences pregnancy outcome. Apparently a minority of scientists believe that it does, while a majority holds the opposite view. The controversy is vividly illustrated by the following exchange of opinions in a leading medical journal. An editorial comment (1) stated that " . . .though pregnant and lactating women deserve special care, the notion that in well fed communities they hover on the brink of undernutrition and even malnutrition stems from lack of knowledge about the metabolic readjustments of pregnancy." The editorial concluded by saying that "in more prosperous societies dietary supplements and nutrition counseling are unlikely to improve fetal outcome." These comments were answered by an irate scientist "aghast at the irresponsibility and incompetence" reflected by the editorial "when discussing the most important health and social problem of our era" (2).

The issue is not a purely academic matter. In the last decade the United States and other countries have spent a considerable amount of money in supplemental food programs for pregnant women. These efforts were motivated by the conviction that such programs would be beneficial but, as indicated by the editorial comments mentioned above, these views are not universally shared. In fact, the mostly negative results of nutrition interventions aimed at improving pregnancy outcome in presumably undernourished women are considered the strongest evidence against the relevance of nutrition and the usefulness of food supplementation during pregnancy.

In recent years new data on the effects of undernutrition on maternal-fetal exchange of nutrients have revealed unexpected facts which challenge some of the old concepts and have shed new light on some of the previous mysteries (3, 4). The overall result has been a much needed revitalization of the field. The purpose of this chapter is to discuss new developments in the field of nutrition and pregnancy and the impact that these new developments have had on some of the most relevant and controversial aspects of the problem. I shall discuss both major concepts and some of the practical issues.

MAJOR CONCEPTUAL ISSUES

Fetal Parasitism

The unique situation of pregnancy has been alternatively described as an harmonious living together of the mother and the fetus (5) or as a period of "physiological stress in which the fetus taxes the maternal organism with its growing needs" (6). The prevailing view, however, is that the mother and the fetus become a new integrated system which, physiologically and metabolically, serves to best meet both maternal and fetal needs. Thus, the present concept is closer to the idea of maternal and fetal symbiosis than the older ideas of "stress" and "competition." Balance and body composition studies support the concept of maternal-fetal biological harmony by demonstrating that under normal circumstances a mother can support normal fetal growth while either maintaining or even increasing her body stores of nutrients (5). The effect of inadequate food intake on maternal-fetal sharing of nutrients is still a matter of controversy. The traditional belief, still held by many, is that "it makes physiological sense for the mother to bear the brunt of the effects of food deprivation" (7). As clearly stated nearly six decades ago, "the fetus lives, like a true parasite, regardless of the expense to the mother" (8).

The opposing view, supported by the most recent data, is that malnutrition prevents the mother from supporting normal fetal growth. As a consequence, although the mother is affected, the fetus is proportionally more affected than the mother (9, 10). This idea was first proposed early this century (11) but it was subsequently forgotten.

The concept of the fetus as a parasite was based on the assumption that the fetal metabolic rate was much faster than the maternal metabolic rate (12). This would allow the fetus to compete metabolically for available nutrients with all maternal tissues except the brain (12). More recent information on fetal oxygen consumption indicates that fetal metabolic rates are higher than maternal rates in some species but either similar or lower in others (13). Hence metabolic competition based on higher fetal rates seems theoretically possible in some species, whereas in others either the mother has an advantage over the fetus or they have equal standing.

The erroneous idea about the fetal capacity to compete with the mother led to the misinterpretation of the results of animal studies. Experiments conducted in rats are a good example. These studies (14) reveal (1) that a severe food restriction is needed to reduce birthweight, and (2) that body weight in the restricted mother is considerably lower than in well-fed control mothers. Both observations apparently support the idea of fetal parasitism since they suggest that the mother has sacrificed her body stores of nutrients to support fetal growth. However, the comparison between well-fed and food restricted pregnant animals may be misleading with respect to the magnitude of the maternal depletion caused by food restriction. Pregnant animals gain a substantial amount of fat which is subsequently lost during lactation. Thus, the differences in body weight of well-nourished and food restricted pregnant animals reflect both what the mother failed to gain and what she has lost to sustain fetal growth. However, if the restricted mother is compared with a nonpregnant animal fed the same quantity of diet for a similar length of time, it becomes apparent that the pregnant restricted rat loses only a minimal quantity of body weight (15). Thus, the food restricted rats are apparently able to protect their nutrient body stores as effectively as nonpregnant animals. They accomplish this by substantially increasing their "food efficiency," defined as the amount of weight gained per gram of food consumed (15). The extra nutrients made available by this mechanism would allow the mother to support fetal growth only to the extent of producing smaller but mostly viable fetuses, without depleting her own prepregnancy stores.

When the food restriction imposed in the pregnant rat is extreme, such as a 75% reduction in food intake, a substantial number of embryonic or early fetal deaths takes place. The final result is a substantial drop in the number of fetuses near term and a 50% reduction in fetal weight. By comparison, maternal body weight is reduced by approximately 32%. Again, the data contrast with the concept of fetal parasitism by showing that in the most extreme conditions not only fetal growth is severely compromised but also fetal survival.

The results of the studies of dietary manipulations suggest that the fetus does not have an unlimited access to maternal nutrient stores. If maternal food intake is inadequate the mother can protect her body stores despite the fact that the fetus becomes growth retarded. The precedence of maternal needs over fetal needs is best illustrated by refeeding experiments carried out in pregnant rats submitted to food restrictions for different lengths of time during gestation. As shown in Table 4-1, if rats are restricted to 25% of their normal intake (75% re-

Table 4.1   Effect of Nutrition Rehabilitation after a Period of 75% Food Restriction on the Mother and the Fetus[a]

	Change in Weight	
Days of Restriction[b]	Mother[c] (%)	Fetus[d] (%)
0	+28	−
5	+27	0
7	+23	− 6.5
9	+21	−12.0
11	+19	−15.5

[a]Adapted from Berg (14).
[b]Since day 1 of gestation.
[c]Maternal weight after removal of uterus and its contents.
[d]Percent change compared with mean birth weight of control fetuses.

striction) between days 1 and 5 of pregnancy, and then fed unrestricted quantities of a normal diet until term (on day 21 of gestation) their final body weights are similar to controls. If the animals are refed only during the last 14 days of pregnancy the mother increases her net body weight by 23% (versus 28% in controls) while the fetuses show a significant 6.5% deficit in body weight. If refeeding is started in the last 12 days the mothers gain 21% net body weight and the fetuses show a significant 12% deficit in body weight. A similar uneven distribution of available nutrients has been observed in rats 50% food restricted between days 5 and 13 of gestation and then refed with either carbohydrate or protein supplements until term (16). The most marked effect was observed in the rats refed with the protein supplements; these animals were able to accumulate 33.6 grams of extra net weight over their initial body weight while the fetuses were still significantly smaller than controls (approximately 11% lighter).

Evidence contrasting with the idea of fetal parasitism can also be found in the available human data. A good example is the study of the effects of the Dutch famine on human development (17).

During the winter of 1944–45, several Dutch cities were exposed to a severe food shortage that lasted approximately 28 weeks. It has been estimated that the per capita caloric intake during that period of time dropped to a low of approximately 1200 kcal/day. Many women were pregnant during the famine and, although it is conceivable that they may have received some extra food from relatives, their food intake must have fallen considerably short of their needs. An analysis of the effects of famine on birth weight revealed a significant decrease of approximately 250 g, compared with prefamine values, for women affected by famine during the second and third trimesters of gestation. This seemingly small difference (approximately 10% of birth weight) caused by conditions considered extreme apparently supports the idea that the human fetus is also an effective parasite or, conversely, that the mother is able to adapt to a reduced food intake to sustain fetal growth.

However, a question that is rarely considered is the effect that pregnancy under famine conditions had on the Dutch mothers. No data have been made available on the prepregnancy weight and changes in body weight of these women. It is, therefore, difficult to establish whether severe food restriction in humans results in changes in maternal body weight and birth weight similar to those described in food restricted rats. However, since the postpartum weight (9–10th day after delivery) of some of the affected Dutch women had been reported (17), it is possible to make some gross estimates of their body weight losses using some reasonable assumptions. The first assumption, considering that the average weight of a young adult female in an industrialized country is 56 kg, is that the average body weight of a fertile Dutch woman during the prefamine period and following many months of food rationing was 55 kg or less. The mean postpartum weight during the prefamine period was 59 kg. Estimating that this weight includes 3 kg due to extra body fluids, enlarged breasts, and enlarged uterus, the women that delivered during the prefamine periods would have gained an average of 1 kg of extra body stores (presumably all fat). If the same factors are subtracted from the postpartum weight of women that suffered famine during various periods of pregnancy it is found that the women most affected by famine may have lost an average of 1.5 kg initial body weight (Table 4-2). Since in this group the reduction in mean birth weight was approximately 10% compared with prefamine values, it is obvious that the mothers affected by the famine were not severely depleted and that they were proportionally less affected than their infants. Thus, in this regard, the human data are consistent with the animal data.

The maternal-fetal division of nutrients during a refeeding period following a severe food restriction has not been studied in humans. Again, some information can be derived from the Dutch famine data (17). This study indicates that when food became available after the fam-

Table 4.2   Estimated Changes in Postpartum Maternal Body Stores and Changes in Mean Birth Weight Caused by the Dutch Famine

Period of Famine	Maternal Weight Postpartum (kg)	Change in Body Stores (kg)	Birth Weight (g)
Prefamine	59.0	+1.0	3338
During 3rd trimester	57.6	−0.4	3220
During 2nd and 3rd trimester	56.5	−1.5	3011
During 1st and 2d trimester	61.0	+3.0	3370
During 1st trimester	61.6	+3.5	3312
Postfamine	62.0	+4.0	3308

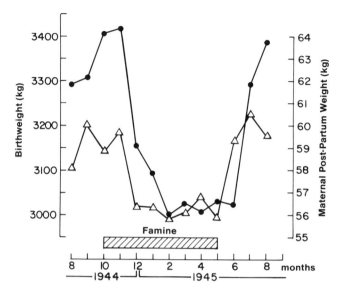

Figure 4-1. Effect of famine on birth weight and maternal postpartum weight in a Dutch population. Adapted from Stein and co-workers (17).

ine, maternal recovery of prepregnant stores, as reflected by maternal postpartum weight increments, preceded the recovery in mean birth weight by approximately 4 weeks (Figure 4-1). This suggests that a certain accumulation of maternal body stores preceded the improvement in fetal growth. A similar phenomenon can be observed in women who start their pregnancy underweight. In these mothers mean birth weight increases proportionally to maternal weight gains during pregnancy but the increments in net maternal weight far exceed those in birth weight (4).

Diet Outcome

Another popular myth in the field of nutrition and pregnancy is the idea that the maternal diet, implying calories and protein intake, can have a direct effect on fetal growth. For example, if a pregnant woman has a lower than average food intake the birth weight of her baby will be lower than average. Conversely, if her food intake is above average the birth weight of her infant also will be above average. Diet quality is also supposed to influence fetal growth but its effect would be less evident than the effect of food intake. These ideas have been the source of much confusion and controversy through the years and they have been equally misused by those who believed in the importance of maternal nutrition and the more numerous skeptics.

The maternal body is not simply a vehicle to make nutrients available to the fetus. Nutrients must be digested, absorbed, transported in the blood, and transferred to the fetus across the placenta. In addition, maternal tissues utilize some of the available nutrients. At each of these various stages problems may develop.

As indicated by refeeding studies in the rat (14) and comparisons of maternal weight gain and increments in mean birth weight in pregravid underweight women (4), when nutrients are made available after a period of food restriction the mother first accumulates weight and then the fetus begins to grow at a faster rate. This indicates that the diet must increase maternal body mass before the fetus can benefit from the available nutrients.

Numerous data on the influence of maternal weight on birth weight indicate that maternal body mass has a profound influence on birth weight. Overweight women tend to have larger infants whereas underweight women tend to have smaller infants (4,18–21). Measurements of food intake in a healthy primigravida population have shown that at midgestation caloric intake is similar in pregravid overweight and underweight women (22). This indicates that during pregnancy women tend to lower their prepregnancy caloric intake if it was high or to increase it if it was low. This convergence toward an average range is also consistent with the observation that overweight women, whose food intake is presumably higher than average, tend to gain less weight during gestation than pregravid underweight women, whose weight gain and caloric intake tend to exceed average values (2).

Observations of the influence of weight gain during pregnancy on birth weight indicate that pregravid obese women who gain little or no weight during pregnancy still deliver infants of average or larger than average size (18–20). Obviously, these women had a low gestational caloric intake. By contrast, pregravid underweight women must gain considerably more weight than average in order to have infants of average or above average birth weight (Figure 4-2). A high weight gain implies a high caloric intake (23). Thus, depending on pregravid maternal weight two strikingly different gestational caloric intakes may result in infants of a similar weight. It is therefore not surprising that caloric intake has little or no correlation with mean birth weight once maternal size is

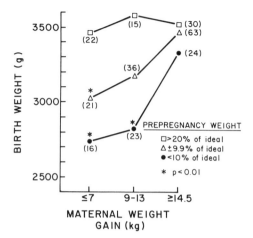

Figure 4-2. Influence of prepregnancy weight and weight gain during pregnancy on mean birth weight at term in 254 low income primiparas and multiparas (4). Numbers in parentheses represent number of subjects.

controlled or held constant (24). In fact, information on maternal caloric intake is absolutely worthless as a predictor of outcome unless adequate data on prepregnancy maternal weight are also considered. As mentioned above, a mother with an "excessive" caloric intake may be an underweight woman trying to reach a normal weight near term. In contrast, a low caloric intake may reflect the reluctance of an obese woman to gain further weight during pregnancy.

A similar criterion can be applied to the influence of diet quality on pregnancy outcome. The possible consequences for the mother or the fetus of unbalanced diets or diets deficient in one or more specific nutrients will depend on the severity of the dietary inadequacy, the maternal nutritional status before pregnancy, and whether the diet is consumed throughout pregnancy or only for a certain period of time (25).

The idea that the quality of the diet has an important influence on birth weight was very popular about 50 years ago (24). Many studies were conducted during that period which showed that vitamin and mineral supplements had a beneficial effect on birth weight (24). Most of these observations did not survive the test of more rigorous studies and, most likely, reflected the presence of uncontrolled confounding variables. For example, a study still quoted in the literature showed a linear correlation between daily maternal protein intake and birth weight (26). Although the importance of an adequate protein intake during gestation is undisputed, the significant correlation found in this study can be explained by the fact that caloric intake and protein intake are highly correlated. Therefore, the observed correlation between protein intake and birth weight can be explained by caloric intake which, in turn, may reflect either maternal body size, or, in a malnourished population, maternal weight gain.

Maternal-Fetal Exchange

Until recently, fetal growth retardation due to maternal undernutrition was attributed to the direct effect of reduced availability of nutrients. Thus, during maternal undernutrition "nutrients circulating in maternal blood are reduced so that the fetus is starved as the mother is" (27).

The possibility that severe maternal undernutrition may affect fetal growth because the plasma levels of critical nutrients fall below critical levels is a plausible one. Metabolic studies in both humans and animals have shown that relatively brief periods of starvation cause a rapid fall in maternal plasma glucose level and a rapid mobilization of lipid as well as enhanced gluconeogenesis (28,29). A prolonged state of semistarvation is likely to perpetuate these changes, causing a reduced availability of glucose and probably key essential amino acids for the fetus. However, the theory of reduced nutrient availability cannot explain the fetal growth retardation associated with suboptimal maternal nutritional status. For example, in developing countries it is common to see women who are moderately underweight as a result of a marginally inadequate food intake. These women are not acutely undernourished and their body weight may remain constant for years. They may have lost weight at one time but then reached a new steady state in which the energy intake is adequate for the metabolic rate of their lower body mass and daily activities. These women may gain 9–10 kg during gestation, allowing them to accumulate some extra body stores, but the average birth weight of their infants is substantially below average, usually slightly above 3000 g, or even less for short women. The situation is analogous to that of the underweight mother in the more affluent countries. These women tend to gain more nutrient stores (or net weight) than the average women; nevertheless, the mean birth weight of their infants remains considerably below average (30) (Table 4-3). In this case there is clearly not a nutrient shortage and nevertheless the fetus does not grow properly.

Table 4.3   Average Net Gain Over Pregravid Weight and Mean Birth Weight in Pregravid Normal and Underweight Women[a]

Group	Number	Net Increase[b] (kg)	Birth Weight (g)
Normal	63	3.2	3400
Underweight	30	4.3	3090

[a]Adapted from Tompkins, Wiehl, and Mitchell (30).
[b]Net increase = postpartum body weight −prepregnancy weight.

The theory of fetal growth retardation due to a reduced availability of nutrients in maternal blood does not then explain the lower birth weight of the infants of underweight mothers. Neither does it explain why maternal accumulation of body stores precedes recovery from fetal growth retardation when undernourished women or animals are refed. Both situations suggest that there are mechanisms limiting the quantity of nutrients made available to the fetus if maternal nutritional status is less than optimal. These mechanisms are not yet fully understood but recent information has provided new and interesting insights into the effects of malnutrition on maternal-fetal exchange.

The fetus has direct access to the nutrients circulating in the maternal blood through the placenta and more indirect access through the amniotic fluid. Circulating nutrients can diffuse into the amniotic fluid and can be swallowed and, eventually, incorporated into the fetal organism. This route of fetal nutrition has been demonstrated in the subhuman primate (31) and it probably also exists in the human fetus. Despite the existence of a transamniotic route of supply, the placenta is the major organ for fetal nutrition. During maternal undernutrition placental growth is reduced and several biochemical alterations, including a shift in the polysomal profile and increased RNase activity, are known to take place (33, 34). Other data suggest that some of the placental hormonal functions, such as estrogen synthesis, may be affected by malnutrition (35). Morphologically, the placentas of malnourished women have a decreased number of villi and a reduced villous surface (36). These changes suggest that the capacity of the placenta to transport nutrients may be reduced by malnutrition. Such a reduction in placental function would explain why the fetus of a malnourished mother seems to have a reduced access to the nutrients available in the maternal body. Studies in malnourished rats have shown that, indeed, the rate of maternal-fetal transfer of nutrients is reduced during maternal malnutrition (37, 38). Nevertheless experiments in vitro demonstrated that the capacity of the rat placenta to incorporate and concentrate amino acids is preserved during malnutrition (39). This fact led to the idea that a reduced blood flow to the placenta might be the main cause for the observed reduction in the maternal-fetal transfer of nutrients. Experiments in food restricted rats later demonstrated that this hypothesis was correct. Animals fed 50% of their normal intake during the course of pregnancy have a marked, approximately 50%, reduction in uterine blood flow near term (40). Hence, while the capacity of the placenta to transfer nutrients may not be altered by malnutrition, less nutrients are made available for transport by a reduced blood flow.

The mechanisms by which maternal malnutrition reduces placental blood flow in the rat have not yet been fully elucidated. It has been shown in the pregnant ewe that the gestational increments in uterine blood flow are closely related to increments in cardiac output (41). Virtually the entire observed increase in cardiac output is destined to accommodate the increased blood flow to the uterus. In food restricted rats cardiac output is approximately half of that of controls; however, the proportion of cardiac output that flows through the uterus is similar to that in controls (40). This fact supports the possibility that the main reason for a reduced uterine blood flow in the malnourished rat is a reduced cardiac output. In the nonpregnant state cardiac output can be increased by a variety of mechanisms. During late pregnancy the major mechanisms seem to be a moderate increase in heart rate and a substantial expansion in blood volume. Experiments in either food restricted or protein restricted pregnant rats have shown that malnutrition substantially decreases blood volume expansion (42). The dampening effect was more evident in the protein deprived animals, suggesting that blood volume expansion is influenced by the availability of essential amino acids.

The studies of plasma volume expansion and uterine blood flow indicate that maternal malnutrition interferes with the normal physiological adjustments of pregnancy. Fetal growth retardation would be the end result of these abnormal changes rather than a direct consequence of a reduced availability of nutrients. This new perspective on the mechanisms of fetal growth retardation would also explain why the mother appears relatively protected in comparison with the fetus. Since fetal growth ultimately depends on uterine blood flow, the failure of the malnourished mother to increase uterine blood flow would also prevent her from making available to the conceptus all the nutrients required for normal fetal growth (3).

Determining whether uterine blood flow is reduced in malnourished women poses obvious technical and ethical limitations. Because of these limitations a more indirect approach has been used to explore the problem. Preliminary results of a study conducted among low income Chilean women show that underweight mothers have a lower plasma volume compared with either average weight or overweight women (43). These preliminary human data support the possibility that the mechanisms described in undernourished animals may also be present in undernourished humans. The findings are not surprising. In nonpregnant subjects it is well established that plasma volume is closely associated with body mass. Nomograms have been made available to estimate plasma volume using body weight and height (44). Since obese women have larger plasma volume than average, and also larger infants, it is tempting to speculate that both factors are associated. Thus, the effect of maternal body weight on birth weight discussed earlier would be mediated by differences in maternal plasma volume and, ultimately, the rate of placental blood perfusion would be indirectly determined by a larger or smaller plasma volume.

MAJOR PRACTICAL ISSUES

Recommended Diet

Because of the lack of adequate metabolic studies or longitudinal studies of food intake in large groups of healthy, well-fed, pregnant women allowed to eat to satisfaction, the present dietary recommendations amount to little more than a series of reasonable guesses.

An urgent need exists for studies of maternal energy requirements. The present recommendations are based on an estimate of caloric costs of pregnancy based on a factorial approach. The value derived from this method amounts to approximately 75,000 kcal or approximately 280 kcal/day over a 40 week period (45).

An attempt to measure the energy needs of pregnant women using indirect calorimetry concluded that the extra metabolic costs of pregnancy amount to approximately 27,000 kcal. This value is very similar to the theoretical estimate (46). Unfortunately, the study was conducted on a captive and nonrepresentative small number of women, some of whom were overweight and had periods of negative energy balance.

As noted above, adequate data on the spontaneous energy consumption of normal free-living women are lacking. A study of 54 middle-class American women measured before and after one or more pregnancies suggests an average pregravid energy intake of approximately 1870 kcal/day and a peak of approximately 1950 kcal/day at midgestation (22). A smaller study in 15 Swedish women, interviewed at the end of each trimester of gestation, also showed a peak of caloric intake at midgestation. Daily caloric intake at this time was 2396 kcal compared to 1980 kcal at the end of the first trimester (47). Many other studies are available on food intake of pregnant women but they do not provide information on gestational changes in intake or there is reason to believe that maternal food intake was influenced by medical counseling or socioeconomic factors. The two studies mentioned above also present problems. In the American women, food intake was probably influenced by the physician's advice. The Swedish study has an inadequate sample size and lacks information about the characteristics of the women to be accepted as representative. Therefore, neither study can be used to assess the extracaloric intake determined by pregnancy. Both studies, however, show an interesting phenomenon, namely, that maternal food intake is maximal at midgestation and decreases thereafter. In the American study daily caloric intake near term is slightly lower than pregravid caloric intake. In the Swedish study no data are available for the last month of gestation but the average caloric intake after the 28th week of pregnancy is 300 kcal lower than at midgestation. A similar pattern can be obtained using a theoretical estimate of pregnancy needs at various times (45). Thus, in contrast with the recommended dietary allowances, which advise a uniform increment throughout gestation, the energy needs of pregnancy are maximal at midgestation. The decline in caloric consumption during the last half of gestation has been attributed to reduced physical activity (48). However, this aspect has never been adequately measured.

The protein needs of pregnant women have been the subject of some controversy. Using a factorial method to estimate protein needs, and assuming a net protein utilization of 70 for the average Western diet, the daily protein requirements would amount to approximately 8.5 g/day (45). However, the current recommendation is 30 g/day (49). The discrepancy reflects the results of nitrogen balance studies conducted in pregnant women, which suggest a much higher nitrogen retention than estimated by the factorial procedure (50). The data were interpreted as indicative of a previously unsuspected maternal protein store. However, more recent nitrogen balance studies have failed to demonstrate the extra nitrogen retention (51), suggesting that the previous data may have reflected overestimation of the nitrogen retained. If the results of these studies are confirmed the current recommendation should be reduced to the previous recommended levels (10 g).

Maternal Weight Gain

The current recommendation is that pregnant women should gain a minimum of 11 kg and, optimally, approximately 12.5 kg. The recommendation derives from a study carried out in a large group of normal Scottish primigravidas (52). This study determined weight gain between the end of the first trimester and term and found it to be 11.4 kg. Assuming a weight gain of 1 kg during the first trimester, the total weight gain of that population was computed as 12.5 kg. This figure has become the recommended ideal.

There is reason to believe that in a general population the average weight gain would be lower than the theoretical 12.5 kg estimate. Although reliable data on changes in body weight during the first trimester of pregnancy are lacking, the fact that most women do not increase their food intake until the end of the first trimester suggests that the estimated gain of 1 kg may be exaggerated. It is also doubtful that a primigravid population would reflect the weight changes of multiparas. Weight gain during pregnancy has been shown to be generally higher in thinner women (19, 20). Women gain weight almost linearly during the third decade of their life, the time when most become pregnant. Therefore, almost by definition, a primigravid, chronologically younger, population should be thinner than a multipara population; hence they would tend to gain more weight. Unfortunately, the available data do not allow one to test the above considerations.

Nearly all studies published to date on weight gain during pregnancy have some limitation, such as small sample size, manipulation of weight gain by health personnel, date of initial measurement not stated, and so on (45). The average weight gain for a multipara population suggested by those studies conducted in affluent countries is approximately 10 kg, computed between the end of first trimester and term.

The use of a recommended weight gain, even if slightly inflated, offers many advantages, since it can be used to monitor progress and to plan nutritional counseling. Unfortunately, the limitations of using such a standard are seldom mentioned. The first and most important limitation is that it applies only to women of average weight and height. In proportion to maternal height the recommendation is too high for shorter than average women and, perhaps, too low for very tall women. More important, the recommendation may be excessive for overweight and obese women and is frankly inadequate for pregravid underweight mothers.

As discussed in detail below more data on normal maternal weight gain are needed and more flexible criteria for weight gain relative to pregravid weight should be established.

Assessment of Fetal Effects

The reduced mean birth weight of the infants of undernourished mothers indicates some degree of fetal growth retardation. As mentioned above, in the Dutch population affected by famine, mean birth weight decreased approximately 327 g, from 3338 to 3011 g (17). This substantial downward shift suggests that most of the infants were growth retarded at birth. However, with the present criteria of growth retardation, only those infants whose birth weight fell below the 10th percentile of a prenatal growth chart would be recognized as being growth retarded. The rest would have been considered normal. This example illustrates the difficulties of recognizing the less severe cases of fetal growth retardation, namely, those infants whose birth weight is still within normal range.

There is evidence indicating that the growth retarding effect of maternal malnutrition becomes apparent only after the 28–30th week of gestation (53). By the 28th week of gestation the average fetus weighs approximately 1200 g, or 2% of the maternal prepregnancy weight, and probably even a moderately undernourished woman can meet the needs of a fetus of this size. However, in the following 10 weeks the normal fetus nearly triples its body weight, thus increasing by a substantial margin its total needs. If the mother cannot meet these needs fetal growth retardation results. The period of rapid fetal body weight increments of the last weeks of gestation coincides with a rapid accumulation of body fat. More than 90% of all the fat present in a normal newborn (approximately 550 g) is deposited during this period (54). A reduced availability of nutrients is likely to interfere with the process of fat deposition. The consequence is reduced weight for length, also reflected in reduced skinfold thickness. This change, analyzed together with the maternal characteristics and pregnancy history, including pregravid weight and gestational weight gain, may indicate whether the infant was affected and, to some extent, the magnitude of the effect.

Depending on the severity of maternal undernutrition, fetal skeletal growth may be retarded. In most cases in which birth weight falls below the 10th percentile of a prenatal growth chart, body length is proportionally reduced. In most of these cases head circumference is also below the 10th percentile. The reduction of head circumference apparently depends on both the severity and the duration of maternal malnutrition. For example, severe malnutrition throughout the entire period of pregnancy would affect all aspects of fetal growth, including head circumference. However, if malnutrition is restricted to the last trimester of gestation, weight and body length could be reduced but head circumference may be normal. These possibilities are still rather tentative since data on the anthropometric characteristics of the infants of undernourished mothers are lacking.

In nonmalnourished women two main types of growth retardation can be recognized: those in which the size of the head is relatively well preserved and those in which the size of the head is reduced proportionally to the rest of the body (52). In the literature these two types of growth retardation have also been called asymmetric and symmetric. These are erroneous names because asymmetry implies different shapes in the halves of the body separated by a sagittal and not a transverse line. Thus, both types of growth retarded infants are symmetric; only the proportion of the size of the head to the size of the body is different.

The two types of fetal growth retardation described have also been observed in laboratory animals and can be induced either by reducing blood flow to the uterus, which causes a disproportionate type, or by malnourishing the mother, which causes a proportionate type (53). In human beings the two types of growth retardation tend to be associated with different maternal conditions, but they also have common maternal conditions (56). Thus, in contrast with earlier assumptions, the two types of growth retardation are not due to different etiological factors.

Ultrasound studies have revealed two major patterns of growth retardation (57). In the first pattern the infant grows normally until the 30th week of gestation, and then there is a sudden reduction in growth rate. The later in pregnancy the onset of growth retardation the less affected the size of the head and also the size of the baby in general. In some of these cases the weight of the baby may be above the 10th percentile despite the retarded ultrasonic growth or it may be below the 10th percentile with a normal ultrasound assessment. Most of these cases of false negative ultrasound diagnosis usually occur when only one ultrasound measurement is made shortly before birth and, therefore, the progressive fall in the rate of increase of the biparietal diameter is not observed. Most of these infants suffer from a disproportionate type of growth retardation.

In the second pattern the infant has been growth retarded since early in gestation, typically before the 20th or 25th week of gestation, and its rate of growth may either parallel the normal curve or fall progressively from normal standards. Most of the infants suffer from a proportionate type of growth retardation.

Approximately 80% of all growth retarded newborns suffer from the disproportionate type of growth retardation, while the rest have a proportionate type (56). The infants with the disproportionate type of growth retardation are more commonly associated with maternal toxemia, essential hypertension, and postmaturity, while the proportionate type of growth retardation is more commonly associated with other congenital anomalies and maternal height under 150 cm. In cases of recurrent antepartum hemorrhage and the antecedent of previous small-for-date infants, the number of proportionate and disproportionate types of growth retardation tends to be similar. These data suggest that infants with a disproportionate type of growth retardation are more likely to be associated with maternal conditions that reduce uterine-placental blood flow, whereas the infants with a proportionate type of growth retardation have a reduced growth potential either because they are genetically small or because of severe growth abnormalities. Both types of growth retardation can be recognized in utero by using head circumference/abdominal circumference ratios (56). In cases of disproportionate growth retardation the ratio is higher than 1 while in the disproportionate type of growth retardation the ratio is usually 1 or smaller than 1.

Data on the anthropometric characteristics of the infants affected by the Dutch famine indicate a marked reduction in body fat, reflected by a reduced body weight/length ratio, a slight decrease in body length, and a proportionally smaller decrease in head circumference (Table 4-4). This type of fetal growth retardation fits the theoretical pattern of late onset, where maternal undernutrition was not either severe enough or prolonged enough to cause brain growth retardation, that is, reduced head circumference. Similar anthropometric changes were found in the infants of underweight women who during gestation failed to gain enough weight to offset their initial weight deficit (58). Thus, a moderate degree of maternal undernutrition causes a disproportionate type of fetal growth retardation. The finding is compatible with the postulated reduced placental blood perfusion.

The problem of assessing the magnitude of the effects on the fetus of maternal malnutrition has also been approached by using a comparison of predicted values derived from maternal characteristics at midgestation and fetal characteristics. By using variables such as amino acid plasma levels, maternal leukocyte energy metabolism, and plasma levels of certain minerals, an equation predicting birth value was developed which correlated significantly with observed birth weight (59). However, the large number of measurements involved and the considerable margin of predictive error make this approach impractical and of little value for individual cases.

Table 4.4 Effect of Acute and Severe Maternal Undernutrition in Previously Well-Fed Women on the Anthropometric Characteristics of the Newborns[a]

	Birth Weight (g)	Body Length (cm)	Body Weight / Body Length	Head Circumference (cm)	Head Circumference / Body Length
Before famine	3290	50.0	65.8	34.4	0.688
At peak of famine	3008	48.9	61.5	34.8	0.711
After famine	3289	49.8	66.0	34.9	0.700

[a]Data from Dutch famine study (17). Values are mean.

At Risk Mothers

Nutritional risk during pregnancy is a vaguely defined term. In the past, three aspects have been considered (1) quality of the diet, (2) quantity of the diet, and (3) maternal body weight. All these aspects, either alone or combined, have been used to identify at risk women in the numerous food supplementation studies conducted during the last four decades. Unfortunately, none of them is adequate.

As discussed earlier, the quality of the diet is very important since inadequacies can lead to specific deficiencies. However, most specific deficiencies are moderate and they do not affect fetal growth. This explains the negative results of the many nutrition interventions in which only vitamins and mineral supplements were distributed (60). During the 1960s and early 1970s the erroneous perception that inadequate protein intake was a major nutritional problem stimulated supplementation programs for pregnant women aimed at ensuring an adequate protein intake (58). Again, most of these attempts failed except for those that succeeded in improving maternal caloric intake in populations where the majority of women had a caloric deficit. In fact, not only have most of the protein supplementation studies failed to produce the expected positive effect on birth weight, but if the protein content of the diet exceeded 18% of total calories the effect on birth weight appears to have been negative (62).

The daily quantity of diet consumed, without due consideration to a series of maternal characteristics that can independently influence food intake and birth weight, is usually a meaningless value. It was mentioned earlier that differences in maternal pregravid weight and weight gain in pregnancy could determine markedly different daily food intakes and mean birth weights. This is extremely important in low-income groups in developing countries, often the subjects of this type of study. These women usually have a much lower stature and body weight than the average European and American woman. When their daily caloric intakes are compared with the recommended allowances they appear to be extremely low. However, if the caloric intake is expressed per kilogram of body weight it becomes apparent that they are only marginally calorie deficient. Unfortunately several supplementation studies in developing countries have used estimates of daily caloric intake as the main criterion for considering the population as being at risk without taking into consideration maternal anthropometric characteristics (63).

Maternal body weight has also been used as an index of maternal nutritional status (63). Obviously this is a very crude parameter since body weight is strongly influenced by height and, in general, women with low body weight are also shorter. Thus, a group of low body weight women is likely to include short women of normal weight for height as well as underweight women.

Other criteria of nutritional risk applied in the past to pregnant women include a previous low-birth weight infant (63). This is obviously an unacceptable criterion since besides undernutrition other maternal conditions are associated with low birth weight.

The most reliable index of nutritional risk is a low pregravid weight. The association between low weight for height at conception and poor outcome was first described almost three decades ago in a population of the Philadelphia Lying-in Hospital (30). This study indicated that severely underweight mothers had a nearly threefold increase in the number of low birth weight infants compared with control women of normal weight for height. A similar association between pregravid underweight and reduced mean birth weight was subsequently reported by others (3, 18–21). These studies also showed that the negative influence of low pregravid weight for height can be neutralized by a large weight gain during pregnancy. A study correlating birth weight with maternal body weight and height near term has shown that mean birth weight increases progressively as maternal body mass increases up to a point at which mean birth weight remains constant despite further increments in maternal body mass (3). The data have been interpreted as indicating the existence of a critical body mass necessary to sustain maximal fetal growth. This critical body mass would be equivalent to 120% of standard weight for height of standard tables. For a woman of average weight and height the critical body mass can be achieved by a 12 kg weight gain. For shorter or taller women the quantity of weight to be gained is, respectively, slightly lower or higher.

The influence of maternal body mass on outcome is probably mediated by the characteristics of the maternal physiological adjustments. As previously discussed, maternal blood volume expansion is a key physiological adjustment for a normal placental blood flow. Maternal plasma volume expansion is strongly influenced by changes in maternal body mass. Underweight gravidas have a smaller plasma volume early in gestation and they fail to reach the plasma volume values of normal women near term (43).

Despite the clear association between maternal body mass and outcome, the correlation between these two variables is not strong enough to allow predictions of outcome in individual cases. This reflects the influence of other maternal characteristics on birth weight. Still, as a single variable maternal body mass (expressed as percent of normal standard) at conception is the best single predictor of low birth weight. Weight for height should be the main criterion for identifying women at risk. Underweight women, together with women of average pregravid weight and height who fail to gain weight early in gestation, should be the only targets of food supplementation programs.

In conclusion, this chapter suggests that many basic concepts and long held beliefs in the field of nutrition during pregnancy should be discarded. They reflect myths and misconceptions resulting from either lack of information or erroneous data interpretation. Unfortunately, these false ideas have created the impression that maternal nutrition is a secondary aspect of prenatal care. The practical consequence of this has been considerable neglect of the field. It is hoped that as more data become available the importance of nutrition during pregnancy will receive appropriate recognition and that editorials such as the one cited in the introductory paragraphs of this chapter become obsolete reminders of the dark ages of an extremely important field.

REFERENCES

1. Maternal nutrition and low birth weight. *Lancet* **2,** 445 (1975).
2. Maternal nutrition and low birth weight. *Lancet* **2,** 704 (1975).
3. P. Rosso, *Am. J. Clin. Nutr.,* **34,** 744 (1981).
4. P. Rosso, *Ped. Ann.,* **10,** 430 (1981).
5. F. E. Hytten and A. M. Thomson, Maternal physiological adjustments, in, *Maternal Nutrition and the Course of Pregnancy,* Washington, D.C. National Academy of Sciences, 1970, p. 41.
6. C. E. Gibbs and J. Seitchick, "Nutrition in pregnancy," in *Modern Nutrition in Health and Disease,* R. S. Goodhart and M. S. Shils, Eds., Philadelphia, Lea & Febiger, 1978, p. 743.
7. E. M. Widdowson, "The Demands of the Fetal and Maternal Tissues for Nutrients and the Bearing of these on the Needs of the Mother to Eat for Two," in, *Maternal Nutrition in Pregnancy—Eating for Two?,* J. Dobbing, Ed., New York, Academic, 1978, p. 1.
8. J. S. Fairbairn, Preface to the study "The Effect of Maternal Social Conditions and Nutrition upon Birthweight and Length," Med. Res. Council, Sp. Rep. Series No. 81, 1924.

9. P. Rosso, "Effects of Maternal Dietary Restriction during Pregnancy on Fetal Growth and Maternal-Fetal Exchange in the Mammalian Species," in, K. S. Moghissi and T. N. Evans, Eds., Nutritional Impacts on Women, Hagerstown, Harper & Row, 1977, p. 49.

10. P. Rosso and C. Cramoy, "Nutrition and Pregnancy," in M. Winick, Ed., Nutrition Pre- and Postnatal Development, New York, Plenum, 1979.

11. N. D. Paton, Lancet **2**, 21 (1904).

12. J. Hammond, Proc. Nutr. Soc., **2**, 8 (1944).

13. F. C. Battaglia and G. Meschia, Physiol. Rev., **58**, 499 (1978).

14. B. N. Berg, J. Nutr., **87**, 344 (1965).

15. S. A. Lederman and P. Rosso, Growth, **44**, 77 (1980).

16. S. A. Lederman and P. Rosso, Am. J. Clin. Nutr., **33**, 1912 (1980).

17. Z. Stein, M. Susser, G. Saenger, and F. Marolla, Famine and Human Development, New York, Oxford University Press, 1975.

18. N. J. Eastman and E. Jackson, Obstet. Gynec. Surv., **23**, 1003 (1967).

19. A. S. Ademowore, N. G. Courey, and J. S. Kime, Obstet. Gynecol., **39**, 460 (1972).

20. J. W. Simpson, R. W. Lawless and A. C. Mitchell, J. Obst. Gynec., **45**, 481 (1975).

21. K. R. Niswander and M. Gordon, The Women and their Pregnancies, The Collaborative Perinatal Study of the National Institute of Neurological Diseases and Stroke, Philadelphia, Saunders, 1972.

22. V. A. Beal, J. Am. Diet. Assoc., **58**, 312 (1971).

23. A. M. Thomson, Br. J. Nutr. **13**, 190 (1959).

24. A. M. Thomson, Br. J. Nutr. **13**, 509 (1959).

25. P. Rosso, and S. A. Lederman, "Nutrition and fetal growth," Adv. Perinat. Med., 1984, (in press).

26. B. S. Burke, V. V. Harding, and H. C. Stuart, J. Pediat., **23**, 306 (1943).

27. H. Schneider and J. Dancis, "Abnormalities of Composition of Maternal Blood, in P. Gruenwald, Ed., The Placenta, Baltimore, University Park Press, 1975, p. 178.

28. N. Freinkel, Israel J. Med. Sci., **8**, 426 (1972).

29. J. E. Tyson, K. L. Austin, and J. W. Farinholt, Am. J. Obstet. Gynecol., **108**, 1080 (1971).

30. W. T. Tompkins, D. G. Wiehl, and R. M. Mitchell, Am. J. Obstet. Gynecol., **69**, 114 (1955).

31. R. M. Pitkin and W. A. Reynolds, Am. J. Obstet. Gynecol., **123**, 356 (1975).

32. J. A. Pritchard, Obstet. Gynecol., **25**, 289 (1965).

33. E. M. Laga, S. G. Driscoll, H. N. Munro, Pediatrics, **50**, 33 (1972).

34. E. G. Velasco, P. Rosso, J. A. Brasel, and M. Winick, Am. J. Obstet. Gynecol., **123**, 637 (1975).

35. L. Iyengar, Am. J. Obstet. Gynecol., **102**, 834 (1968).

36. E. M. Laga, S. G. Driscoll, and H. N. Munro, Pediatrics, **50**, 24 (1972).

37. P. Rosso, J. Nutr. **107**, 2002 (1977).

38. P. Rosso, J. Nutr., **107**, 2006 (1977).

39. P. Rosso, Fed. Proc. 250 (1980).

40. P. Rosso and R. Kava, J. Nutr., **110**, 2350 (1980).

41. J. F. Clapp, *Am. J. Obstet. Gynecol.,* **130,** 419 (1978).

42. P. Rosso and M. R. Streeter, *J. Nutr.,* **109,** 1887 (1979).

43. P. Rosso, A. Arteaga, A. Foradori, P. Lira, G. Grebe, P. Vela, and J. Torres, "Plasma volume expansion during pregnancy in underweight normal and overweight low income Chilean women." (In preparation).

44. J. F. Dagher, J. H. Lyons, D. C. Finlayson, J. Shamsai, and F. D. Moore, *Adv. Surg.,* **1,** 69 (1965).

45. F. E. Hytten and I. Leitch, *The Physiology of Human Pregnancy,* Oxford, Blackwell Scientific, 1971.

46. K. Emerson, Jr., B. N. Saxena, and E. L. Poindexter, *Obstet. Gynecol.,* **40,** 786 (1972).

47. N. O. Lunell, B. Persson, and G. Stersky, *Acta Obstet. Gynecol. Scand.,* **48,** 187 (1969).

48. R. N. Taggart, Cited by F. E. Hytten and J. Leitch, *The Physiology of Human Pregnancy,* Oxford, Blackwell Scientific, 1971.

49. Committee on Dietary Allowances, Food and Nutrition Board, Recommended Dietary Allowances, Washington, D.C., National Acad. Sci., 1980.

50. J. C. King, D. H. Calloway, and S. Margen, *J. Nutr.* **103,** 772 (1973).

51. F. D. Johnstone, *J. Nutr.,* **111,** 1884 (1981).

52. A. M. Thomson and W. Z. Billewicz, *Br. Med. J.,* **1,** 243 (1957).

53. P. Gruenwald, "The Supply Line of the Fetus," in, P. Gruenwald, Ed., *The Placenta,* Baltimore, University Park Press, 1975, p. 1.

54. E. E. Ziegler, A. M. O'Donnell, S. E. Nelson, and S. J. Fomon, *Growth,* **40,** 329.

55. P. Rosso and M. Winick, *J. Perinat. Med.,* **2,** 147 (1974).

56. A. Kurjak, V. Latin, and J. Polak, *J. Perinat. Med.,* **6,** 102 (1978).

57. S. Campbell, "Physical Methods of Assessing Size at Birth," Ciba Foundation Symposium 27 (New series), 275, 1974.

58. P. Rosso, A. Arteaga, A. Foradori, P. Lira, G. Grebe, P. Vela, and J. Torres, "Maternal Nutritional Status and the Outcome of Pregnancy in Low Income Chilean Women," 1983. (In preparation).

59. J. Metcoff, J. P. Costiloe, W. Crosby, L. Bentle, D. Seshachalam, H. H. Sandstead, C. E. Bodwell, F. Weaver, and P. McLain, *Am. J. Clin. Nutr.,* **34,** 708 (1981).

60. L. Bergner and M. W. Susser, *Pediatrics,* **46,** 946 (1970).

61. B. Chow, A. M. Hsueh, and R. Q. Blackwell, "Taiwan Study," in *Nutritional Supplementation and the Outcome of Pregnancy,* Washington, D.C., National Acad. Sci., 1973, p. 111.

62. D. Rush, "Effects of Changes in Protein and Calorie Intake during Pregnancy on the Growth of the Human Fetus," in J. Chalmers and M. Enkin, Eds., *Effectiveness and Satisfaction in Antenatal Care. Clinics in Developmental Medicine Series,* London, Spastic International Med. Publ., 1982, p. 95.

63. D. Rush, Z. Stein, and M. Susser, "Diet in Pregnancy: A Randomized Controlled Trial of Nutritional Supplements," *Birth Defects,* original article series, **XVI** (3), 1980.

5

Nutrition and Brain Development

MYRON WINICK, M.D.

Institute of Human Nutrition, Columbia University College of Physicians and Surgeons, New York, New York

Even before the turn of the century it was well known that children who suffered a severe bout of undernutrition early in life grew poorly, if at all. What was unclear until much later was whether if food subsequently became available these children would reach normal height. Two schools of thought existed, one asserting that severe undernutrition early in life resulted in permanent growth stunting and the other claiming that with proper rehabilitation these children could recover and ultimately reach their normal height.

In the early 1950s the now classical experiments of Kennedy, McCance, and Widdowson settled the disagreement and demonstrated that both schools were right. These investigators malnourished two groups of rats. Both groups were still growing, but one was malnourished from birth to weaning (21 days) whereas the second group was malnourished after weaning. The results were quite clear. In the first group the animals were small at the end of the period of malnutrition and remained stunted no matter how they were subsequently refed. By contrast, in the second group the animals were also smaller at the end of the period of malnutrition but after adequate refeeding these animals caught up and attained their normal size.

Thus these experiments identified a key variable in determining whether recovery from early malnutrition could occur. The variable was time. The experiments had demonstrated that there was a fundamental difference between early growth and later growth which allowed the animal to recover when malnourished later but precluded such recovery when the malnutrition occurred earlier. And yet careful assessment of growth by the methods available at that time (length, height, tail length, and various other anthropometric measures) could not determine what that fundamental difference was.

It was not until 1964 that two investigators, Enesco and LeBlond, at McGill University, began to shed light on this problem. They were working on what appeared to be a totally different question. What they were asking was, as any organ grows or increases in size, is it because the number of cells is increasing or because the size of already present cells is getting larger, or is it for some combination of these reasons? It had already been determined that DNA, the genetic material, was found almost exclusively in the cell nucleus and that in any species the amount of DNA in a diploid nucleus was constant. That is, every rat diploid cell contained the same quantity of DNA as every other rat diploid cell, and all human diploid cells contained the same amount of DNA. For many species the constant had already been determined, for example, 6.2 pg per rat diploid cell and 6.0 pg per human cell. Thus by determining the total DNA content in the various organs of the rat and dividing by 6.2 pg they could determine the number of cells in any organ at any time. Once the number of cells had been determined, these investigators could divide that number into the total weight of the organ and determine an average weight per cell; or they could divide that number into the total protein content of the organ and determine an average protein content per cell. If we wish only to *compare* changes in cell number or cell size we can express the data as total organ DNA (reflecting cell number) and weight/DNA or protein/DNA, reflecting average weight per cell or total protein per cell, an indication of cell size. Using these measurements Enesco and LeBlond asked a very simple question, how do the organs of the rat normally grow as the rat increases its size with maturity? Figure 5-1 demonstrates their results.

The normal period during which the organs of the rat increase in size is from the early prenatal period to 120 days after conception (100 days after birth). However the number of cells (DNA content) reaches a maximum long before growth stops. The time at which this maximum is reached will vary from organ to organ. In the brain and lung maximum cell number is reached at about 21 days after birth and in the heart at about 65 days after birth, but in every case before growth stops. Hence there must be a period of growth when the organ is enlarging but the number of cells is not increasing. The size of the cells is getting larger.

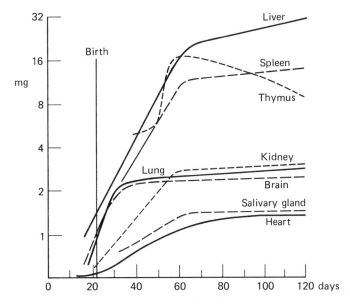

Figure 5-1.   DNA content of various organs.

Subsequent studies revealed that there are actually three phases of growth undergone by all organs. During the first phase total organ DNA increases and organ weight or protein increases *at the same rate*; hence the ratio does not change. Cell number is increasing while cell size is remaining constant (hyperplasia). During the second phase cell number continues to increase but at a slower rate than before. Total weight and protein content continue to increase at the same rate as previously; hence the weight/DNA and protein/DNA ratios begin to increase. Both cell number and cell size are increasing (hyperplasia and hypertrophy). During the third phase of growth cell number is no longer increasing, weight and total protein continue to increase, only cell size is enlarging (hypertrophy).

From these data it became clear that by measuring changes in cellularity a fundamental difference between early growth which was hyperplastic and later growth which was hypertrophic could be defined. Was this the fundamental difference uncovered by the British investigators ten years previously and did this difference explain the recovery or lack of recovery in the two groups of animals they had studied? A series of experiments in the late 1960s answered these questions. The results demonstrated that when undernutrition occurred during the period of hyperplastic growth, the rate of cell division was slowed, resulting in a smaller organ with fewer cells. Since the time during which cells divide is fixed, this change was permanent if the rehabilitation took place after that time had elapsed. By contrast, if the undernutrition occurred during the period of hypertrophy the normal increase in cell size was prevented. However, with subsequent rehabilitation the cells just filled back up with protein and attained their normal size.

These data also demonstrated something else. The number of cells in any organ at any time is not simply a function of genetics. The environment acting at a critical time, namely, the period of hyperplasia, could influence the rate of cell division and ultimately the final number of cells. Other experiments demonstrated that such alterations could be induced in either direction. Thus overfeeding rats from birth to weaning resulted in a larger animal, with larger organs composed of an increased *number* of cells. These studies have subsequently been expanded by focusing on the adipose tissue and have had a major impact on our understanding of obesity.

The knowledge that permanent organ stunting could be induced by early undernutrition and that the stunted organ contained fewer cells raised some important questions relating to the growth of the brain.

By the time these experiments became known, other investigators had determined that early malnutrition affected brain growth by retarding the rate of myelination. And yet another group of scientists were demonstrating behavioral abnormalities in animals undernourished during the first 21 days of life—abnormalities that persisted into adulthood. Thus the effects of early malnutrition on brain structure and function were already being studied. Theoretically both reduced myelination and abnormal behavior might be explained by a reduction in brain cell number, particularly in specific brain regions. Experiments examining cellularity in various brain regions of rats who had been subjected to early malnutrition were therefore undertaken.

Results of these experiments can be summarized as follows. In the rat the most rapid rate of cell division postnatally was found in cerebellum, and it stopped at about 14 days of age. In cerebrum the increase was slower but continued longer, to 21 days of age. And in brain stem there was a very gradual increase which lasted only until the 14th day of life. In addition, in the hippocampus (an area concerned with certain emotions) there was a very discrete increase between the 14th and the 16th day. This increase was shown to be due to a migration of neurons from

under the lateral ventricle into the hippocampus which occurred pre-
cisely on the 15th day. Thus, in determining the effect of early postnatal
undernutrition on the cellularity of various brain regions it became important to assess the effects on cell migration as well as on cell division.
Such experiments were undertaken and revealed that the earliest and
most severe effects were on cerebellum. After only 8 days of
undernutrition beginning at birth, a reduced cell number could be demonstrated in that region. By contrast it took 14 days of undernutrition
beginning at birth to produce any effect on cerebrum. Undernutrition
beginning at birth and continued for the first 21 days of life also prevented the migration of cells from under the lateral ventricle into the
hippocampus. These studies were the first to demonstrate what subsequently turned out to be a general principle. It made no difference what
region of the brain was being studied. What was important was the rate
of cell division in that region. The more rapid the rate of cell division the
earlier and the more profound the effects of malnutrition.

Studies in which maternal malnutrition was induced throughout
pregnancy demonstrated an even more profound effect on brain
cellularity, and combined prenatal and postnatal malnutrition produced
the most serious reduction in cell number.

By this time it had become important to try to determine which cell
types (primarily neurons or glia) were affected by early malnutrition.
For these experiments the technique of radioautography had to be used
since total DNA analysis could not differentiate one cell type from another. By using this technique it was shown that only glial cells were dividing postnatally in rat cerebrum and that undernutrition reduced the
rate of cell division among these cells. In cerebellum the internal granular, the external granular, and the molecular cells, all primitive neurons,
were still dividing and undernutrition impeded their rate of cell division. Finally, the primitive neurons under the third and lateral ventricles
were still dividing and undernutrition retarded their rate as well. Since
the latter cells would migrate to the hippocampus on the 15th day of life
it was felt that this migration was prevented by reducing the number of
cells at the source. These studies suggested another general principle.
The type of cell was unimportant; what mattered was whether that cell
was dividing at the time the malnutrition was imposed. This suggestion
was further strengthened by experiments in which radioautography was
performed after prenatal malnutrition had been imposed and the fetal
brain was examined on the 16th day of gestation. The results demon-

strated that in every area studied both glial and neuronal cell division were impeded.

Although research was still continuing very rapidly with experimental animals (by this time dogs, pigs, and subhuman primates, as well as rats, were being studied) a number of studies were also being conducted in human populations. These studies were suggesting that early malnutrition, particularly infantile marasmus, would result in permanent behavioral abnormalities which were reflected by reduced IQ scores and poor school performance. Therefore in the early 1970s a series of studies were undertaken to determine whether severe early malnutrition could result in changes in the cellular growth of the human brain which were similar to those found in animals. Before such studies could be undertaken, however, it was important to determine the pattern of cell division in the normal human brain. To that end a study was carried out on the brains of infants who had died of accidents, poisonings, or crib deaths, and on the brains of fetuses from therapeutic abortions due to psychiatric problems in the mother. The results of this study (Figure 5-2) demonstrated that the number of cells in the human brain increased linearly during prenatal life and then began to level off around the time of birth. By 18 months of age cell number has reached adult

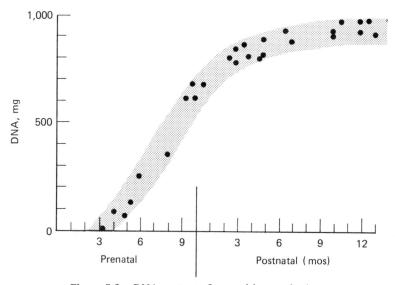

Figure 5-2. DNA content of normal human brain.

levels. Thus there is no increase in cell number in the human brain after 18 months of age. Since brain weight and total protein content increase until beyond 3 years of age, all growth after 18 months is due to an increase in cell size. Other studies subsequently carried out by Dobbing and Sands have indicated that two major spurts of cell division take place in the human brain. The first occurs in early prenatal life (around the fourth month of gestation) and is primarily due to the proliferation of neurons. The second occurs around the time of birth and is primarily due to the proliferation of glia. When the regional pattern of cell division in the human brain was studied it was found that the most rapid rate of cell division in the human brain postnatally was in cerebrum and that in cerebrum, cerebellum, and brain stem cell number reached its maximum at about 18 months of age. From these studies it was expected that the kind of malnutrition in the human that was most likely to retard the rate of cell division was severe undernutrition beginning in utero or shortly after birth. For this reason studies were undertaken in infants who died of severe marasmus during the first year of life. These studies were carried out in Santiago, Chile. The results demonstrated a reduced DNA content in the brains of these marasmic infants (Figure 5-3). The reduced DNA content in whole brain was reflected by a reduced DNA

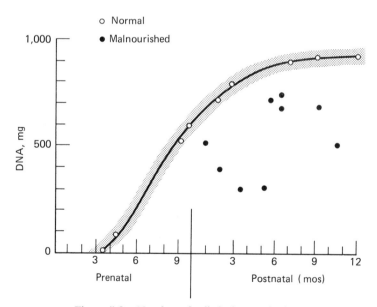

Figure 5-3.   Number of cells in human brain.

content in cerebrum, cerebellum, and brain stem. Thus early severe malnutrition beginning in the first year of life, and severe enough to cause death resulted in retarded cell division in the human brain. This retardation was found in all three regions of the brain that were studied. By this time it was already known from animal experiments that severe early malnutrition affected the rate of myelination of the brain and reduced the content and concentration of several of the gangliosides in brain tissue. Studies in these infant brains revealed similar changes. The total brain cholesterol content (one measure of total myelination) was reduced in the infants who died of marasmus. The total brain phospholipid content (another measure of total myelination) was also reduced in these infants. The lipid to DNA ratio, which reflects the amount of myelin per cell, was normal in infants who died in the first 6 months of life and was reduced in infants who died later. This would indicate that malnutrition during the first 6 months of life reduced myelination and cell number proportionally. If the malnutrition persisted beyond 6 months the reduction in myelin exceeded the reduction in cell number, since myelination normally continues for a much longer period of time than cell division. These data in humans were exactly the same as what had been previously described in rats and pigs. In addition, studies on these human brains revealed that both ganglioside content and concentration were reduced. Gangliosides are lipoprotein complexes that are present almost exclusively around the dendrites near the synaptic junctions. Reduction in their content suggests a reduced number of synapses. Reduction in their concentration suggests that the reduction in synapses is greater than the reduction in brain weight, myelination, or cell number. Again these data confirmed what had been previously found in rats and pigs.

In humans it is also possible to make some measurements in vivo which reflect brain growth. Most important among these is head circumference. By plotting changes in head circumference against total brain weight, total brain protein content, and total brain DNA content, a characteristic pattern emerged. In both normal and malnourished children head circumference could be shown to reflect all of these parameters. Thus severe early malnutrition retarded the growth of the brain and this growth retardation was directly reflected in a reduced head circumference.

Since early malnutrition had been shown to retard the rate of cell division in brain and since the most rapid rate of cell division in that organ is before birth, studies were undertaken to examine the effects of prenatal malnutrition on the developing brain. When the maternal diet was reduced to 50% of control values rats gave birth to pups that were reduced in size and whose brains were smaller and had a reduced number of cells. Other experiments in rats demonstrated that prenatal and postnatal malnutrition resulted in a 50% reduction in brain cell number, more than the combined effect of malnutrition at either period alone.

Studies in human populations had also suggested that prenatal malnutrition alone would retard fetal growth. During the infamous Dutch Hunger Winter of 1945 birth weight was reduced by 250 g. During the siege of Leningrad it dropped by about 400 g. In malnourished populations in some of the developing countries birth weight is about 450 g lower than in more affluent, better nourished populations. In one such population in Guatemala supplementation with 20,000 extra calories throughout the course of the pregnancy resulted in a return of birth weight to normal. Finally, in infants who had died of postnatal malnutrition and who in addition were of low birth weight the number of brain cells was reduced to 50% of normal, which is very similar to the reduction produced in rats by combined prenatal and postnatal malnutrition.

Thus by the middle 1970s it was quite clear that early malnutrition, whether prenatal or during the first 6 months of life, would result in retarded brain growth which was reflected by changes at the cellular level involving a reduction in cell number, a reduced quantity of myelin, and fewer dendritic arborizations. Malnutrition beginning at conception and continuing throughout the first six months of life will cause a profound reduction in cell number. These changes are reflected by a proportional reduction in head circumference. From animal experiments it would appear that these changes are permanent.

At the same time that these studies on early malnutrition and brain cellularity were being carried out a number of investigations of early malnutrition and brain function were underway. Stoch and Smythe in South Africa had studied IQs of children who had been malnourished in infancy and had compared them to IQs of previously well-nourished children. They found a significantly lower mean IQ in the previously malnourished group. However their work was criticized in that the two groups studied were significantly different in many ways other than their early nutritional status. For example, the control children came from better environments, better housing, families with jobs, parents with higher levels of education, and so on. From this study it was not possible to separate the contribution of early nutrition from the contribution of other early environmental influences. This problem has plagued subsequent investigations and even though there has been considerable refinement in methodology over the years, the question of whether early malnutrition *alone* could affect subsequent behavior was not answered until recently. For this reason, a series of animal experiments were undertaken. In these experiments malnutrition was usually induced from birth and extended throughout the nursing period. Since the animals were being nourished by their mother's milk entirely, a number of methods were employed to reduce the quantity of milk produced. These included increasing the number of pups nursing from a single mother (usually to 18), malnourishing the mother, and tying off several of the mother's teats. All of these methods interfered with the normal maternal-infant interaction, a problem that was to have important significance later. Regardless of the method employed, the pups showed a variety of behavioral abnormalities at the time of weaning and these abnormalities persisted into adult life. Hence early malnutrition in these experiments was thought to affect an animal's ability to explore its environment and to negotiate a variety of mazes. In addition the pups were described as hyperactive. In dogs severe early malnutrition could result in a convulsive disorder.

In the meantime several studies in human populations were attempting to control the environment for variables other than early undernutrition. Two of the most important of these studies were carried out in Mexico and in Jamaica. The study in Mexico correlated a variety of social factors with subsequent IQ scores. While the degree of undernutrition and the time it occurred were always important, other factors, such as the level of the mother's education, the ability of the family to contact the outside world, and the father's occupation, were independently related to the outcome. In the study in Jamaica, children who were severely malnourished early in life were compared with siblings and with children of the same age and in the same grade who were from similar social backgrounds but who did not have a history of early undernutrition. The results were very clear. The previously malnourished children consistently had the lowest IQ scores. The siblings were next and the matched controls uniformly did best. These data suggested that early malnutrition may not have been the only factor affecting the subsequent behavior of these children (since the siblings who were not malnourished did worse than the control group). Other types of behavior were also affected. For example, when the teachers were asked "which child in your class is the most difficult to teach?," they consistently picked the child who had been previously malnourished. Similarly, when the child nearest the previously malnourished child in age was asked, "who is the most difficult child to get along with?," again the previously malnourished child was picked. Thus something about the behavior of the previously malnourished child over and above the IQ deficit was affected.

Ten years ago then, although a great deal had been learned about the effects of early malnutrition on the developing brain, the question whether early malnutrition alone could affect subsequent behavior had not been answered.

In the early 1970s a series of experiments in animals began to shed light on this question. The experimental psychologists noted that when animals were reared in isolation from the normal stimuli during early life they showed behavioral abnormalities later in life which were almost identical to those produced by early malnutrition. Levitsky and Barnes postulated that perhaps there was an interaction between early nutrition and early environmental isolation which resulted in the behavioral abnormalities. They reasoned that perhaps early malnutrition functionally isolated the animal from its environment and in that way resulted in the behavioral deficits. To test their hypothesis they studied four groups of rats. One group was isolated from their environment but normally nourished; the second group was isolated from their environment and simultaneously undernourished; the third group was undernourished but received environmental stimulation by being handled for 5 minutes three times a day; and the fourth group was normally nourished and stimulated in the same way. The results of behavioral tests were very clear. The isolated malnourished animals did the worst. The stimulated normal animals did the best and the performance of the isolated normal and the stimulated malnourished was in between. From these results it was clear not only that early nutrition and early environment interacted but that environmental stimulation could prevent some or all of the behavioral abnormalities previously ascribed to early malnutrition. Subsequent experiments in animals strongly supported this concept. Frankova, in a series of experiments performed in the United States and in Czechoslovakia, demonstrated that by placing a virgin female rat that had been previously trained to take care of pups (which she called an aunt) in the cage with a malnourished mother and her pups, the expected behavioral consequences were averted. The aunt, by stimulating the pups, had allowed them to develop normally even in the face of early malnutrition.

Studies in human populations also were suggesting that an interaction between early malnutrition and the overall poor environment in which this malnutrition was taking place was responsible for the subsequent behavioral abnormalities. Children with cystic fibrosis, who were every bit as malnourished as the children from developing countries in the studies, but who had grown up in a stimulating environment, were shown to have normal IQs when studied after reaching school age. Children born during the Dutch Hunger Winter, whose mothers had been severely malnourished during pregnancy and who themselves were underweight at birth, had perfectly normal IQs when studied 20 years later. While these studies suggested that environmental enrichment might be able to prevent the effects of malnutrition in children whose malnutrition did not occur under the usual poverty conditions, they did not directly answer the question whether children malnourished under the conditions prevalent in developing countries could benefit from subsequent environmental enrichment.

To answer this question two studies were done with Korean orphans. In the first study three groups of children were investigated. In the first group the children had been severely malnourished in the first 6 months of life. In the second group they were moderately malnourished, whereas the children in the third group were well nourished during the first 6 months of life. All of the children were adopted by middle-class American families before they were 3 years old. The children were examined for IQ score and school performance between ages 10 and 12. The IQs of the previously severely malnourished children averaged 103. The previously well-nourished children had IQs averaging 112, and the IQs of the previously moderately nourished children were in between (Figure 5-4). When school performance was examined the results were similar. The previously malnourished children were performing right at stanine 5, which is the U.S. norm, whereas the previously well-nourished children were performing significantly above that norm. Again those children who had been moderately undernourished during the first 6 months of life were performing in between. These data demonstrated that although differences could still be demonstrated between children who were severely malnourished in the first 6 months of life and those whose nutrition at that time was normal, these differences were very

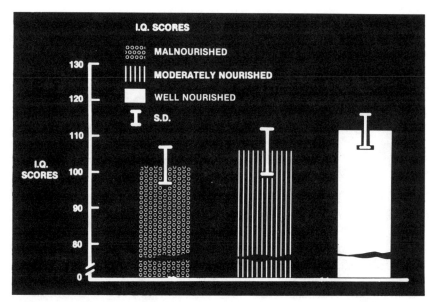

Figure 5-4. IQ scores in three groups of Korean orphans adopted before age 3.

small by the time the children reached age 10–12, if a stimulating environment was introduced before the child was 3 years old. In addition, the degree of recovery under these conditions was very impressive. Previous studies had repeatedly shown that children malnourished under similar conditions, if subsequently returned to the environment that produced the malnutrition, would have average IQ scores 25 or 30 points below the scores achieved by the children in this study. An important question, however, remained unanswered. How early does environmental enrichment have to be started to obtain these results? To answer this question a similar study was conducted, except that all of the children were adopted between ages 3 and 5. The results showed a drop in IQ and performance in all three groups (Figure 5-5). The previously malnourished group was now performing significantly below U.S. norms. But even in these later adopted children there was significant recovery when compared to the results to be expected if these children had been returned to the original environment that had led to the malnutrition. When all of the children in the two studies were compared using time of adoption as the main variable it became clear that there was a linear inverse relationship between time of adoption and subsequent performance. The later the adoption the poorer the outcome. A

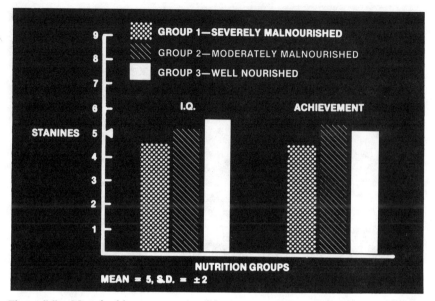

Figure 5-5. IQ and achievement scores of three groups of Korean orphans adopted after age 3.

final study, investigating the relationship of early environment and poor nutrition to subsequent behavior, was carried out in the United States. It was assumed that children raised in a single foster home would be subjected to a more stable environment than children who were moved from foster home to foster home. When two such groups were compared, the mean IQ score of those raised in multiple foster homes was 14 points lower than the mean IQ of those raised in single foster homes. These data, of course, did not prove cause and effect, since it was quite possible that families receiving children with low IQs were more likely to reject them. However this interpretation became less likely when one correlated the height of the children in both groups with the outcome. In the single foster home group there was no correlation. By contrast, in the multiple foster home group there was a strong correlation. The shorter the child the lower the IQ. Since short stature is one of the known consequences of severe early malnutrition these data suggest an interaction of early nutrition and early environment in determining subsequent outcome.

Hence the data in both animal experiments and human studies suggest a complex relationship between early undernutrition and subsequent behavior. This relationship involves an interaction between the malnutrition and the whole poverty cycle, an interaction that somehow results in permanent developmental retardation. This interaction, while necessary for the behavioral effects, is not necessary for the cellular effects.

Very recent studies have attempted to seek a biochemical mechanism for the behavioral effects. One component of gangliosides, n-acetyl neuraminic acid (NANA), is reduced in the brains of animals subjected to early malnutrition by the usual methods but unaffected when these animals are stimulated simultaneously. Environmental stimulation alone will increase cerebral NANA concentration. Labeled NANA injected intraperitoneally shows rapid incorporation into brain gangliosides during the first 28 days of life, with little incorporation thereafter. Repeated injections of NANA during the first 28 days of life will prevent the behavioral changes in malnourished animals and raise the brain NANA levels to the same degree as environmental stimulation. Although these data do not prove that reduced NANA levels are the mechanism mediating the interaction of environmental isolation and early malnutrition, they suggest that a chemical basis for this interaction may exist.

It is clear that during the past 20 years much has been learned about early undernutrition and subsequent brain development. From a structural standpoint the brain can be permanently altered by early malnutrition *alone*. From a behavioral standpoint it appears that the early malnutrition must be accompanied by environmental deprivation in order for permanent consequences to ensue. Present research is focusing on the biochemical basis for this early interaction between undernutrition and environmental isolation. Perhaps in the next 20 years this complex interaction will be understood. Until then it is crucial that early malnutrition and the poverty cycle that produces it be eliminated for the sake of the next generation of children.

SUGGESTED READING

M. Winick, *Malnutrition and Brain Development*, New York, Oxford University Press, 1976.

M. Enesco and C. P. LeBlond, *J. Embryol. Exp. Morph.* **10,** 530 (1962).

M. Winick and A. Noble, *Devel. Biol.,* **12,** 451 (1965).

M. Winick, *Pediat. Res.,* **2,** 352 (1968).

J. Dobbing and J. Sands, *Arch. Dis. Child.,* **48,** 757 (1973).

E. M. Widdowson and R. A. McCance, *Proc. Roy. Soc. London,* **152,** 88 (1960).

A. N. Davison and J. Dobbing, *Br. Med. Bull.,* **22,** 40 (1966).

S. Zamenhof, E. Van Marthens, and L. Grauel, *Science,* **174,** 954 (1971).

M. Winick and P. Rosso, *Pediat. Res.,* **3,** 181 (1969).

P. Rosso, J. Hormazabal, and M. Winick, *Am. J. Clin. Nutr.,* **23,** 1275 (1970).

D. A. Levitsky and R. H. Barnes, *Nature,* **224,** 468 (1970).

J. Cravioto, E. R. DeLicardie, and H. G. Birch, *Pediatrics,* **38,** 319 (1966).

Z. Stein, M. Susser, G. Saenger, and F. Marolla, *Science,* **178,** 708 (1972).

D. A. Levitsky and R. H. Barnes, *Science,* **176,** 68 (1972).

M. Winick, K. K. Meyer, and R. C. Harris, *Science,* **190,** 1173 (1975).

M. L. Nguyen, K. K. Meyer, and M. Winick, *Am. J. Clin Nutr.,* **30,** 1734 (1977).

M. Winick, A. Jaroslow, and E. Winer, *Growth,* **42,** 391 (1978).

6

Thermogenesis in Human Obesity

F. XAVIER PI-SUNYER, M.D.

St. Luke's-Roosevelt Hospital Center and Columbia University College of Physicians and Surgeons, New York, New York

In recent years, there has been renewed interest in possible thermogenic differences between lean and obese subjects. It has been suggested that the obese may be more "efficient;" that is, that they may require fewer calories for energy maintenance and thus require fewer calories per unit of lean body mass or of weight. If such were the case, since energy balance implies an equilibrium between energy expenditure and energy intake, they would require fewer calories to maintain a given weight. The evidence for and against this will be reviewed in this chapter.

Energy expenditure is made up of three components, basal metabolic rate, activity, and the thermic effect of food. The basal metabolic rate has been operationally defined as the calories expended per unit time by a relaxed person who is in a thermoneutral environment and who has been fasting for 12 to 18 hours. The calories expended for a particular activity can be calculated as those calories utilized above the caloric cost of basal metabolism. The thermic effect (TEF) of food has been previously called the specific dynamic action (SDA) and is defined as the elevation of metabolic rate occurring after food ingestion.

In this chapter, I will discuss in turn each of these three components, asking the question, Is there a difference between the lean and the obese in this expenditure? I will confine myself essentially to data in the human and refer the reader to other excellent reviews of thermogenesis in small animals.

BASAL METABOLIC RATE

The basal metabolic rate (BMR) defines that energy which is necessary for the basic maintenance of the body. This includes energy used for the movement of the heart and muscles, for maintenance of ionic gradients between cells and the body fluids for synthesis of new protein, and for maintenance of the body temperature. Also some energy is used up as a result of the inefficiency of doing the above work.

As mentioned above it has been suggested that the obese are overweight because they are hypocaloric. To discuss this hypothesis, the units of measurement of BMR must first be defined. A measurement of kilocalories of energy per unit of time allows for calculation of total expenditure of an organism per hour or per day. It stands to reason that the energy needed to maintain a small organism, say a rat, will be less than that needed to maintain a large organism, such as a man. In order to try to compare energy expenditure of different sized animals, gross total expenditures per unit time have been divided into an equalizing or standardizing measure. Height, weight, surface area, or lean body mass have been used as the denominator for such a correction. If energy was expressed per unit of weight, however, it was early noted that metabolic rate decreases as animals increase in size. Weight, therefore, is not a good standardizer. Surface area has been used because it tends to equalize better than weight does the energy expenditure between different sized organisms. But normalizing energy expenditure in relation to surface area is essentially inaccurate, because it does not account for differences in body composition. Although surface area does reduce variation caused by differences in body size, a better relationship can be obtained by relating energy expenditure to lean body mass (1). By such a transformation, one can compare energy expenditure of different groups; better still, one can also compare different individuals of the same group.

Standardization of BMR by lean body mass (or fat-free mass, FFM) has been widely advocated (2–4). Such standardization by lean body mass eliminates the diminution of BMR seen with age (2,5,6). Since the studies just referred to dealt with normal weight individuals, it was unclear how such data would apply to overweight ones. Of the studies that have been done in this regard, some suggest that BMR in the obese is best related to lean body mass (7–9), others to fat mass (10), and some to both (11). We (12) studied 154 obese women and 49 obese men before the beginning of a weight reduction program and found that the contribution of the FFM to the BMR was three to five times greater per kilogram than that of body fat. Since we found no significant difference in regression coefficients between men and women, we postulate that the difference in BMR between the sexes is caused by the higher lean body mass in males.

In general, others have also found that lean body mass correlates best with basal metabolic rate. It explains why men have higher metabolic rates than women and why metabolic rates decrease with age. The much higher metabolic rate of children can be explained by the energy cost of growth (13, 14).

Why Bray and co-workers (10) found a much greater effect of body fat than FFM on BMR is puzzling. Two factors may help to account for this finding. First, many of their measurements were after meals. Second, they studied 13 extremely fat women. Possibly, the extremely large adipose mass in these patients made it quantitatively more important than lean body mass as a determinant of BMR; also, it is possible that the method for measuring lean body mass on these very obese patients was inappropriate (1).

However, comparing individuals of the same group by using a normalizing ratio such as lean body mass may be misleading. In thinking about caloric expenditure and energy balance, we are really interested in total energy flow in and total flow out, and this is usually more instructive than expressing the data over a denominator, whatever that denominator may be.

Boothby and co-workers (15) showed that, even with very careful measurements, there was still a very great variation in the rate of energy expenditure between individuals. Even when subjects were matched for age, sex, and surface area, a coefficient of variation of 9% was found. Such a ±9% coefficient, however, does not define the limits of normality of expenditure of an individual. Warwick and co-workers (16), for instance, have shown differences in metabolic rate of more than 30% in individuals of the same age, sex, weight, and life-style.

If we can agree that there is a difference in metabolic rate among individuals, and that this can be as high as one-third of total calories expended, then it is clear that, at a given caloric intake, one individual might gain weight and one might not. It follows from this that energy balance depends on matching intake to expenditure, and that it is not surprising that different individuals will maintain weight on widely differing caloric intakes.

Since basal metabolic rate is very difficult to measure, resting metabolic rate is most often used by investigators in the laboratory. This is usually done with the individual lying in a thermoneutral environment, having fasted for 8 hours, and having abstained from all activity for a period of at least one half hour. The individual is as unstressed as possible but is not asleep. The minimal energy expenditure can be measured about 4 or 5 AM during an individual's overnight sleep. It is then about 10% lower than under basal conditions (17). However, Durnin and Passmore state; "in our experience, rates of resting energy expenditure obtained just before rising reflect accurately the rate of expenditure during the whole period in bed" (18).

It has been generally found that the BMR of the obese is higher than that of the lean (19–24). Also, in overfeeding studies, the BMR rises as weight is gained (25). Thus, there is little argument in the literature against the notion that obsese persons expend more total energy than leans. It is also known that obese subjects have a greater lean body mass than leans (21, 22). This is because they require a certain extra amount of sustaining cell mass to maintain the extra fat. It is most likely because of the larger lean body mass that BMRs are higher in the obsese. However, when their BMR is expressed relative to body weight, the obese often have values below the leans. This is because per unit of weight they may have a relatively lower amount of metabolizing cell mass in relation to the amount of body weight (17). The decreasing BMR per kilogram of body weight as body weight rises was documented by Keys and Brozek (26).

In summary, it seems reasonable to compare basal metabolic rates of obese and lean as actual total amount of energy per unit time (minute, hour, day) or as energy per unit time per unit of lean body mass (or fat-free mass). When either of these measures is used, the overwhelming evidence suggests that the obese expend more calories than the lean. In terms of basal or resting energetics, therefore, no case can be made for the statement that the obese are hypocaloric and more efficient than the lean.

THE THERMIC EFFECT OF FOOD

Food is a very important thermogenic stimulant since as it is metabolized it causes heat production. Because of this, a fed animal has a higher metabolic rate than a fasting one. This elevation of metabolic rate above basal after eating has been called the thermic effect of food (TEF) or dietary induced thermogenesis (DIT). The increase in heat production was originally called the specific dynamic action of food and was attributed to protein. We now know that carbohydrate and fat also have heat producing effects, though not to the same degree that protein does (27–29). With a mixed diet, about 10% of the metabolizable energy ingested is lost as heat. This heat is used in the intermediary metabolism of substrates, in the utilization of ATP, and in the formation of ATP from reduced coenzymes by oxidative phosphorylation.

Since the thermic effect of a meal is small, it is difficult to measure accurately. A control day in which food is not given is required to observe in a given individual what is truly heat production from the meal and what is the normal diurnal rise in oxygen consumption. While, as mentioned above, the increase in oxygen consumption following a meal averages about 10% above baseline, there may be rhythmical variations of baseline, unrelated to food, of up to 20% over a 24-hour period (30) and variations also occur in an individual from day to day.

Although a number of studies have been done on the thermic effect of food in the obese and lean, many are technically suspect. Four early studies suggested a reduced thermic effect of food in obese subjects (31–34). Kaplan and Leveille (35) studied the calorigenic response to a semisynthetic 823 kcal high protein test meal in adult women with a history of childhood onset obesity. They reported that the obese have a lower thermic effect of food than the lean. However, inspection of their data shows a statistically significant difference when actual oxygen consumption increases are compared. Significance is detectable only if the oxygen consumption is expressed in terms of body weight to the 0.75 power. The fallacy of such a ratio has already been discussed.

Shetty and co-workers (36) studied five lean, five obese, and five reduced obese subjects, giving them a liquid mixed meal of 9.8 kcal/kg of ideal body weight. They found a smaller increment from baseline in O_2 consumption in obese than in lean. They found a significantly decreased increment in the reduced obese also. However, if one calculates the total energy expended during the meal, since the basal rate of the obese was significantly higher, in fact the obese were expending a greater total energy during the meal than the lean. The significance of this study is therefore unclear.

Pittet and co-workers (37) gave 50 g of glucose to six lean and six obese women and reported a thermic effect of the food that was 13%

above baseline in leans and only 5% above in obese. This is a technically excellent study.

In contrast to these three studies, there are others that suggest no difference in the thermic effect of food between leans and obese. Lauter (38), Strang and co-workers (39), Clough and Durnin (40), and Cunningham and co-workers (41) found no such thermic effect difference of mixed meals.

With regard to carbohydrate loads, neither Sharief and McDonald (26) nor Welle and Campbell (42) agree with Pittet (37). Sharief and McDonald (24) studied five obese and six lean individuals, by giving them orally 5 g/kg of ideal body weight of glucose and sucrose. For a 3-hour period O_2 consumption and CO_2 production were measured and no difference was noted between leans and obese in the thermic effect of either carbohydrate. Welle and Campbell (42) studied 11 leans and 13 obese women after 100 gm of glucose orally and saw no difference in the thermic effect over baseline in obese as compared to leans. They suggest that possibly Pittet and co-workers studied obese subjects with an impaired glucose tolerance so that all glucose may not have been utilized over 3 hours and it is for this reason that they may have obtained a smaller thermic effect in the obese.

Rothwell and Stock (43) have suggested that insulin is required for a full diet-induced thermogenic effect in the rat. It certainly seems possible that insulin deficiency or insulin resistance could lead to defective glucose oxidation and thus to impaired thermogenesis. This could explain why some studies of carbohydrate feeding in obese showed a decreased thermogenic response (37) and other studies did not show such a decreased response (24, 42). In an important study, Golay and co-workers (44) measured 55 nondiabetic and diabetic obese and 30 nondiabetic volunteers. They found that postprandial thermogenesis induced by the oral glucose was decreased in the presence of insulin resistance or reduced insulin response.

Other evidence for the importance of adequate insulin biological activity for maximal thermogenesis has come from the study of Thiebaud and co-workers (45). They studied 22 healthy young volunteers with a euglycemic glucose clamp technique whereby they could maintain blood glucose level constant while raising the insulin by graded levels from 62 to 1132 μU/mL. They found that glucose oxidation increased as insulin levels rose from 62 to 103 to 170 μU/mL and then reached a plateau at levels above 170 μU/mL.

Thus, these studies suggest that insulin is required for adequate carbohydrate oxidation and that whether an obese individual has an impaired thermogenic response to a carbohydrate meal may depend less on his obesity per se and more on the level of insulin resistance or insulin deficiency that he manifests.

It is my conclusion that the evidence for a diminished thermic effect of food in obese humans as compared to leans is meager. Certainly this is so in studies using mixed meals. For each study showing such a response, there are two not documenting it. Also, even in those studies showing a decreased thermic effect in the obese, if this TEF is added to the resting metabolic rate, the overall energy expenditure in the obese is greater than in the lean for a period of 3 or 4 hours after a meal.

It is likely, based on the most recent studies, that some thermogenic defect relating to carbohydrate ingestion may be found in obese who are insulin resistant and not found in subjects who are equivalently obese but are insulin sensitive. It is obvious that investigators in the future will have to distinguish between types of obesity and degrees of glucose intolerance when doing studies of the thermic effect of food.

THERMOGENESIS AND OVERFEEDING

The term "luxus consumption" was coined 81 years ago by Neumann (46) to describe his own ability to maintain a specific weight while eating different amounts of calories. He postulated that when he overate, he wasted the extra calories as heat, and thus maintained his weight stable without conscious effort. Since that observation, there has been continuing controversy over whether with overfeeding there is an increased heat production so that a significant amount of energy is wasted rather than stored, both at rest and during activity.

Garrow (47) has summarized the results of 15 studies (25,46,48–60) in which subjects were overfed. In reviewing the studies, certain conclusions may be reached. First, the BMR was raised by overfeeding in all the studies measured, except that of Glick and co-workers (60). Unexplained heat losses, that is, greater energy expenditure than could be accounted for from the measurements of metabolic rate, activity expenditure, and estimated energy stores from weight gain, were reported by seven studies. Of these seven, only four really provide evidence against energy wasting (49, 52, 54, 60). As Garrow (47) says, "The remaining publications either directly support the idea of some form of luxus consumption or provide data which are difficult to understand unless some such mechanism exists."

In the four studies not showing an energy wastage effect, either the overfeeding was for less than 2000 cal per day or had been carried out for less than 10–12 days. Thus it may be that a critical amount of overfed calories may be necessary for a critical amount of days before the "luxus consumption" phenomenon occurs.

Once having concluded that there is quite good evidence to suggest that with significant overfeeding (of the order of 2000 extra calories per day) for a sufficient length of time (about 10 days) energy wastage occurs, how do we relate this to leanness and obesity?

In the 15 studies reviewed above, 57 subjects were initially lean and 23 were obese. In the four studies in which obese subjects were studied, no evidence of luxus consumption was found. Does this mean that leans are able to burn off excess energy while obese are not? More comparative studies in the same laboratory are necessary to evaluate this. However, one fact is clear from the data of Goldman and co-workers (25)—that the numbers of calories required to maintain a previously lean individual at an overweight level is much higher than that required to maintain an already obese individual at the same overweight level. The reason for this is unclear, but it does suggest increased efficiency of at least some obese subjects.

In the studies of Sims and co-workers (25, 61–63), the increased thermic effect of overnutrition appeared as an increment in the basal or resting oxygen consumption (63). These investigators concluded that although a wastage effect occurred, it was small, of the order of 15% of the BMR. As Danforth and co-workers (63) state, these changes in thermogenesis "test the limits of sensitivity of the methods used to assess the changes and may account for some of the disagreement in the literature on this subject." They go on, "It is tempting to speculate that, if normal people react to overfeeding by using some of the calories inefficiently, spontaneously obese people may lack such a protective mechanism against obesity. However, there is no convincing evidence to date in the literature that there is a lack of this sort in any of the syndromes of obesity."

It must also be kept in mind that instances of calorie wastage have been documented only with extremely large calorie overloads. No evidence exists for any effect of smaller loads in either lean or obese. Thus, the experimental data described above cannot be invoked to postulate that a lean woman overeating 300 calories or so per day might have an energy wastage that would allow her to keep weight at equilibrium, while an obese woman overeating the same 300 calories, would not waste them as heat and as a result would gain weight. This has not been shown in either lean or obese subjects.

No systematic studies have been done comparing overfeeding of the same number of calories to lean and obese subjects over protracted periods of time and calculating accurately the total energy spent and documenting whether this energy expenditure is greater than when smaller amounts of calories are eaten.

It is true that there is a great deal of evidence in small rodents for the luxus consumption phenomenon. Under cafeteria feeding (64) or with high sucrose diets (65) rats will overeat and, though they will gain weight, all of the calories overeaten cannot be accounted for by the enhanced energy reserve deposited as fat. There is a definite ability of small animal species (mice and rats) to burn off excess eaten energy and stave off obesity to some extent. The wastage of energy seems to be mediated through activation and hypertrophy of brown adipose tissue in these animals (66). Brown adipose tissue, activated by the sympathetic nervous system, can greatly enhance its activity and produce much greater amounts of heat (67–69). Although the mass of brown adipose tissue is small, even in the hypertrophied state, Foster and Frydman (70) have shown that blood flow through the brown fat can be greatly enhanced and can account for the increased thermic release observed in small animals.

A deficient ability to burn off excess calories has been documented in a series of genetically obese rodents (71). The activation of thermogenesis has been tested by placing obese animals in cold environments and documenting whether the liberated norepinephrine will enhance thermogenesis and maintain temperature. Defective thermogenesis has been documented in the *ob/ob* mouse (72, 73). It has also been documented in the *db/db* mouse (74). Such thermoregulatory defects have also been documented in the yellow obese mouse and the Zucker fatty (*fa/fa*) rat (75).

However, whether wastage of energy with overfeeding occurs in man has already been discussed and whether, if it does, defective activation of such thermogenesis occurs in obese adults is unclear. There is very serious doubt whether an adequate amount of brown fat exists in adult man to mount the excess heat production required. Although some brown fat activation by norepinephrine has been documented in man (66) the quantitative significance of this is not at all clear. Jung (76) has shown a defective thermogenic response to norepinephrine in obese and reduced obese subjects, but Daniels and co-workers (77) could not duplicate this in fat Pima Indians on a weight maintenance diet. Therefore, whether even a norepinephrine insensitivity occurs in obese man is unclear.

The extrapolation of small animal data to man is not warranted at this time. The final question is whether in response to usual environmental stimulants at believable stimulatory levels, the obese will respond with lower energy expenditure than the lean. The stimulants one can invoke are food, cold, stress, and exercise. We have already discussed food. Cold is unlikely to be a stimulant because in our society people do not voluntarily suffer cold but cover and protect themselves from such discomfort. Stress is difficult to study because it is hard to quantitate and reliably duplicate in separate trials; as a result, no adequate studies have been done. Exercise, however, needs to be discussed.

THERMOGENESIS DURING FOOD AND EXERCISE

Several investigators have studied whether an additive increase in the thermogenesis induced by food occurs when exercise is introduced, or whether more than expected or less than expected energy expenditure occurs. Also, some have tried to document whether the response is different in leans and obese.

These are difficult studies to do, as Garrow intimates (47), because the differences to be measured are very small and to obtain reliable data, an experimenter must do four studies for each determination—without food or exercise, with food, with exercise, and with food and exercise. As the baseline changes from day to day and changes during the study (30,42) a large number of trials and subjects must be used to obtain reliable data. As a result, one must read some of the published data very critically.

Some have tested only leans (78–82); others have tested only obese (83,84). A few have tested both lean and obese (60,85,86). In the study of Bray and co-workers (81), six normal weight subjects exercised by pedaling a stationary bicycle which allowed for variable resistance. The volunteers were given both 1000 and 3000 kcal breakfasts or no breakfast at all. Exercise after breakfast was associated with a higher oxygen uptake than without breakfast. This was true even when a correction was made for the thermic effect of the breakfast itself. However, both caloric loads gave the same results. Bray concluded that food intake increases the energy expended during muscular contraction by 5 to 10%, independent of the thermic effect of food itself.

Other studies have suggested a similar enhancement. Miller and coworkers (78) found a doubled thermic effect of food when light exercise was added (but the observations were few). Bradfield and co-workers (83) also showed such a potentiating effect. Unlike Bray, however, when they gave a greater caloric load they obtained a greater potentiating effect.

In contrast to the above three studies, which showed a potentiating effect of exercise on food thermogenesis, there are a greater number that do not show such a phenomenon. Swindells (79) could demonstrate no potentiating effect in lean subjects and neither could Hansen (80) or Warnold (82). Apflebaum (84) could not find it either in obese subjects.

Glick and co-workers (60) studied both lean and obese women whom they initially kept at maintenance weight or then overfed for 5 days by 2300 calories above their weight maintenance period. They found no increase in energy expenditure to a given bicycle ergometer task when subjects were either overfed or normally fed as compared to the energy expenditure in the unfed state. This was true of both obese and lean subjects.

Strong, Shirley, and Passmore (54) also compared the effect on thermogenesis in lean and obese who were overfed for 4 days and exercised. The study was less controlled than Glick's (60) in that they allowed a wide range of variability both in excess intake and in expenditure, so that the leans overate more and exercised less than the obese. Nevertheless, their results were similar to Glick's in showing no effect of activity in increasing dietary thermogenesis during the overfeeding period.

Zahorska-Markiewicz (85) studied the thermic effect of food and exercise in 10 lean and 14 obese women. She had her subjects eat a 1000 kcal mixed content meal and then exercise or not exercise following the meal. The exercise consisted of 60 watts of an electrically braked bicycle ergometer. The experiment is flawed in that neither a no exercise nor a no exercise-no food trial was run. Nevertheless, the data showed that while there was an increment of food plus exercise that was close to additive in the leans, the obese showed no added expenditure of food plus exercise over just exercise, suggested a "saving" of calories in the obese that was not found in the lean.

Segal and Gutin (86) tested energy expenditure on a bicycle ergometer in 10 lean and 10 obese women with similar lean body mass but different fat mass. They tested them with a work load set at each individual's anaerobic threshold, and at rest. The subjects were tested after eating a 910 kcal mixed meal and again without the meal. An equivalent thermic effect of the meal alone was found in both the lean and the obese women. On addition of exercise, a potentiating effect of food by exercise was seen which was modest, but statistically significant. The elevations in the exercise metabolic rate were 12.1% and 10.6% for the lean group and 4.9% and 3.6% for the obese group at the two levels of exercise. Thus, eating prior to exercise augmented the energy cost of the total period of exercise (40 minutes over 4 hours) by 20 kcal for the lean group and 8 kcal for the obese. The difference in potentiating effect between lean and obese found in this well-conducted study is therefore very small indeed and approximates the error of the methods of measurement even in the most careful hands.

In summary, if there is a potentiating effect of exercise on the TEF, it seems to be very small. It is extremely difficult to demonstrate because very small changes in exercise effort from one trial to the next may cause a larger change in energy expenditure than the change that might be expected in the TEF as influenced by the exercise. It may be that no answer to this question will be found until more accurate methods are available to control exercise energy expenditure or to measure that expenditure. One thing is certain; if a potentiating effect exists it is very small, and if a difference is present between lean and obese, it is smaller still.

Blaza (87) in recent work with Garrow (88) has made a strong case against the notion that obese people are less thermogenic than leans not only to food, but to other stimuli. She studied five lean and five obese subjects in a direct calorimeter for five 24-hour periods each. One was a control day and the other four test days were (1) extra food (800 kcal), (2) exercise (8 miles on a bicycle ergometer), (3) heat (27°C), (4) cold (23°C). Conditions were otherwise similar and the trial days were randomized. Patients were on a 3.4 mJ per day diet. The obese women expended about 60 mL O_2/min more than the lean during the control day and their heat loss was about 37 watts more. Values did not change significantly to either cold, warmth, or food. There was a slight increase of O_2 consumption with exercise, but the 37 watts difference between lean and obese did not change. Thus, in no experimental condition did the energy expenditure of the lean subjects exceed that of the obese.

The authors conclude, "These results suggest that, at least in subjects on a restricted calorie intake, thermogenic responses to ordinary stimuli are small, and do not support the hypothesis that a failure in thermogenic responsiveness is an important factor in the etiology of human obesity" (88).

There seems to be little experimental evidence that there is a difference in lean humans as opposed to obese in wasteful energy production to any stimulant. There are two exceptions to this. First, it is possible that with very great overfeeding (2000 kcal or more above usual intake) for a long period of time (10 days or more) some wasteful energy production will occur and that this may be greater in lean than in obese. Second, it is possible that obese patients with insulin resistance or insulin deficiency may have a specific defect of glucose oxidation and generate less heat after eating carbohydrate than lean or obese individuals with normal insulin physiology.

One should be careful in extrapolating to man thermogenic data collected in rodents. The two organisms may be considerably different in thermogenic activation. Although data for thermoregulatory defects in obese animal models are firm, their extrapolation to man is presently unwarranted. Outside of the two conditions outlined above, no strong data are available for the notion that obese humans are more efficient than leans in the utilization of energy, thereby directing more calories to reserves. Obviously, the matter is controversial, and more careful and well-designed studies are required.

REFERENCES

1. J. S. Garrow, *Energy Balance and Obesity in Man*, 2nd ed. Amsterdam, New York, Oxford, Elsevier, 1978.
2. A. Keys, H. L. Taylor, and F. Grande, *Metabolism*, **22,** 579 (1983).
3. A. T. Miller and C. S. Blyth, *J. Appl. Physiol.*, **5,** 311 (1953).
4. A. R. Behnke, *Ann. N. Y. Acad. Sci.*, **56, 1095** (1953).
5. S. P. Tzankoff and A. H. Norris, *J. Appl. Physiol.: Respirator. Environ. Exercise Physiol.*, **43,** 1001 (1977).

6. J. J. Cunningham, *Am. J. Clin. Nutr.,* **33,** 2372 (1980).

7. W. P. T. James, J. Bailes, H. L. Davies, and M. J. Dauncey, *Lancet,* **1,** 1122 (1978).

8. D. Halliday, R. Hesp, S. F. Stalley, P. Warwick, D. G. Altman, and J. S. Garrow, *Int. J. Obesity,* **3,** 1, (1979).

9. H. Ljunggren, D. Ikkos, and R. Luft, *Br. J. Nutr.,* **15,** 21 (1961).

10. G. Bray, M. Schwartz, R. Rozin, and J. Lister, *Metabolism,* **19,** 418 (1970).

11. M. Hoffmans, W. A. Pfeiffer, B. L. Grunlach, H. G. M. Nijrake, A. J. M. Oude Ophnis, and J. G. A. J. Hauvast, *Int. J. Obesity,* **3,** lll (1979).

12. R. S. Bernstein, J. C. Thornton, M. U. Yang, J. Wang, A. M. Redmond, R. N. Pierson, F. X. Pi-Sunyer, and T. B. Van Itallie, *Am. J. Clin. Nutr.,* **37,** 595 (1983).

13. D. J. Millward and P. J. Garlick, *Proc. Nutr. Soc.,* **35,** 339 (1976).

14. B. W. Spady, P. R. Payne, D. Picou, and J. C. Waterlow, *Am. J. Clin. Nutr.,* **29,** 1073 (1976).

15. W. M Boothby, J. Berkson, and H. L. Dunn, *Am. J. Physiol.,* **116,** 468 (1936).

16. P. M. Warwick, R. Toft, and J. S. Garrow, *Int. J. Obesity.,* **2,** 396 (1978).

17, J. R. Flatt, in G. A. Bray, Ed., *Recent Advances in Obesity Research,* II, London Newman, 1978, p. 211.

18. J. V. G. A. Durnin and R. Passmore, *Energy, Work and Leisure,* London, Heinemann, 1967.

19. J. S. Garrow, P. M. Warwick, S. E. Blaza, and M. A. Ashwell, *Lancet,* **1,** 1103 (1980).

20. F. Grande, *Am. J. Clin. Nutr.,* **21,** 305 (1968).

21. W. P. T. James and P. Trayhurn, *Br. Med. Bull.,* **37,** 43 (1981).

22. E. Ravussin, B. Burnand, Y. Schutz, and E. Jequier, *Am. J. Clin. Nutr.,* **35,** 566 (1982).

23. R. S. Shwartz, J. B. Haler, and E. Bierman, *Metabolism,* **114,** (1983).

24. N. N. Sharief and I. MacDonald, *Am. J. Clin. Nutr.,* **35,** 267 (1982).

25. R. F. Goldman, M. F. Haisman, G. Bynum, E. S. Horton, and E. A. H. Sims, in G. A. Bray, Ed., *Obesity in Perspective,* Vol. 2, Washington, D.C. U.S. Govt. Ptg. Office, 1975.

26. A. Keys and J. Brozek, *Physiol. Rev.,* **33,** 245 (1953).

27. R. B. Bradfield and M. H. Jourdan, *Lancet,* **2,** 640 (1973).

28, J. S. Garrow and S. F. Hawes, *Br. J. Nutr.,* **27,** 211, (1972).

29. S. Welle, U. Lilavivat, and R. Campbell, *Metabolism,* **30,** 953 (1981).

30. J. Aschoff and H. Pohl, *Fed. Proc.,* **29,** 1541 (1970).

31. F. Rolly, *Deutsche Med. Wochenschr.,* **417,** 887 (1921).

32. R. Plaut, *Deutsche Arch. F. Klin. Med.,* **139,** 285 (1922).

33. C. C. Wang, S. Strouse, and A. D. Saunders, *Arch. Int. Med.,* **34,** 573 (1924).

34. E. H. Mason, *Northwest Med.,* **26,** 143 (1927).

35. M. L. Kaplan and G. A. Leveille, *Am. J. Clin. Nutr.,* **29,** 1108 (1976).

36. P. S. Shetty, R. T. Jung, W. P. T. James, M. A. Barrand, and B. A. Callingham, *Clin. Sci.,* **60,** 519 (1981).

37. P. Pittet, P. Chappuis, K. Acheson, F. de Techtermann, and E. Jequier, *Br. J. Nutr.,* **35,** 281 (1976).

38. S. Lauter, *Deutsch Arch. F. Klin. Med.,* **150,** 315 (1926).

39. J. M. Strang and H. B. McClugage, *Am. J. Med. Sci.*, **182,** 49 (1931).

40. D. P. Clough and J. V. G. A. Durnin, *J. Physiol.*, **207,** 89P (1970).

41. J. Cunningham, M. Levitt, R. Hendler, E. Nadel, and P. Felig, *Clin. Res.*, **30,** 244A (1982).

42. S. L. Welle and R. G. Campbell, *Am. J. Clin. Nutr.*, **37,** 87 (1983).

43. N. J. Rothwell and M. J. Stock, *Metabolism*, **30,** 673 (1981).

44. A. Golay, Y. Schutz, H. U. Meyer, D. Thiebaud, B. Churchod, E. Maeder, J. P. Felber, and E. Jequier, *Diabetes*, 31, 1023 (1982).

45. D. Thiebaud, E. Jacot, R. A. DeFronzo, E. Maeder, E. Jequier, and J. P. Felber, *Diabetes*, **31,** 957 (1982).

46. R. O. Neumann, *Arch. Hyg.*, **45,** 1 (1902).

47. J. S. Garrow, in G. A. Bray, Ed., *Recent Advances in Obesity Research*, Vol. 2, London, Newman, 1978, p. 200.

48. A. Gulick, *Am. J. Physiol.*, **60,** 371 (1922).

49. R. Passmore, A. P. Meiklejohn, A. D. Dewar, and R. K. Thow, *Br. J. Nutr.*, **9,** 20 (1955).

50. G. V. Mann, K. Teel, O. Hayes, A. McNally, and D. Bruno, *New Eng. J. Med.*, **353** 349 (1955).

51. N. Ashworth, S. Creedy, J. N. Hunt, S. Mahon, and P. Newland, *Lancet*, **2,** 685 (1962).

52. R. Passmore, J. A. Strong, Y. E. Swindells, and N. el Din, *Br. J. Nutr.*, **9,** 20 (1955).

53. D. S. Miller and P. M. Mumford, in M. Apfelbaum, *Energy Balance in Man*, Paris, Masson, p. 195.

54. J. A. Strong, D. Shirling and R. Passmore, *Br. J. Nutr.*, **21,** 909 (1969).

55. E. A. H . Sims, R. F. Goldman, C. M. Gluck, E. S. Horton, P. C. Kelleher, and D. W. Rowe, *Trans. Assn. Am. Phys.*, **81,** 153 (1968).

56. J. V. G. A. Durnin and N. Norgan, *J. Physiol. Lond.*, **202,** 106, (1969).

57. M. Apfelbaum, J. Bostsarron, and D. Lacatis, *Am. J. Clin. Nutr.*, **24,** 1405 (1971).

58. B. J. Whipp, G. Bray, and S. N. Koyal, *Am. J. Clin. Nutr.*, **26,** 1284, (1973).

59. J. S. Garrow and S. Stalley, *Proc. Nutr. Soc.*, **34,** 84A (1985).

60. Z. Glick, E. Shvartz, A. Magazanik, and M. Modan, *Am. J. Clin. Nutr.*, **30,** 1026 (1977).

61. R. L. Burse, R. F. Goldman, E. Danforth, Jr., E. S. Horton, and E. A. H. Sims, *Fed. Proc.*, **36,** 546 (1977).

62. R. L. Burse, R. F. Goldman, E. Danforth, Jr., D. C. Robbins, E. S. Horton, and E. A. H. Sims, *Am. Physiologist*, **20,** 13, (1977).

63. E. Danforth Jr., A. G. Burger, R. F. Goldman, and E. A. H. Sims, in G. A. Bray, Ed., *Recent Advances in Obesity Research.*, II, London, Newman, 1978, p. 229.

64. N. J. Rothwell and M. J. Stock, *Proc. Nutr. Soc.*, **39,** 45A (1980).

65. J. G. Granneman and G. N. Wade, *Metabolism*, **32,** 202 (1983).

66. N. J. Rothwell and M. J. Stock, *Nature*, **281,** 31 (1979).

67. B. A. Horwitz, *Fed. Proc.*, **38,** 2170 (1979).

68. D. G. Nicholls, *Biochim. Biophys. Acta.*, **549,** 1 (1979).

69. J. Himms-Hagen, *Ann. Rev. Physiol.*, **38,** 315 (1976).

70. D. O. Foster and M. L. Frydman, *Can. J. Physiol. Parmacol.*, **56,** 110 (1978).

71. W. P. T. James and P. Trayhurn, in R. F. Beers and E. G. Barrett, Eds., *Nutritional Factors: Modulating Effects on Metabolic Processes*, New York, Raven, 1981, p. 123.

72. P. L. Thurlby, and P. Trayhurn, *Br. J. Nutr.*, **39,** 397 (1978).

73. P. L. Thurlby and P. Trayhurn, *Br. J. Nutr.*, **42, 377 (1979).**

74. P. Trayhurn and L. Fuller, *Diabetologia,* **19,** 148 (1980).

75. P. Trayburn and W. P. T. James, in B. Cox et al., Eds., *Thermoregulatory Mechanisms and Their Therapeutic Implications*, Basel, S. Karger, 1979, p.251.

76. R. T. Jung, P. S. Shetty, W. P. T. James, M. A. Barrand, and B. A. Callingham, *Nature,* **279,** 322 (1978).

77. R. J. Daniels, H. L. Katzeff, E. Ravussin, J. S. Garrow, and E. Danforth, Jr., *Clin. Res.*, **30,** 244A (1982).

78. D. S. Miller, P. Mumford, and M. J. Stock, *Am. J. Clin Nutr.*, **20,** 1223 (1967).

79. Y. E. Swindells, *Br. J. Nutr.*, **27,** 65 (1972).

80. J. J. Hansen, *J. Appl. Physiol.*, **35,** 587 (1973).

81. G. A. Bray, B. J. Whipp, and S. N. Koyal, *Am J. Clin. Nutr.*, **23,** 254 (1974).

82. I. Warnold and R. A. Lenner, *Am. J. Clin. Nutr.*, **30,** 304 (1977).

83. R. B. Bradfield, D. E. Curtis, and S. Margen, *Am. J. Clin. Nutr.*, **21,** 1208 (1968).

84. M. Apfelbaum, J. Bostsarron, and D. Lacatis, *Am. J. Clin. Nutr.*, **24,** 1405 (1971).

85. Zahorska-Markiewicz, *Eur. J. Appl. Physiol.*, **44,** 231 (1980).

86. K. R. Segal and B. Gutin, *Metabolism*, **32,** 581 (1983).

87. S. E. Blaza, Thermogenesis in Lean and Obese Individuals, Ph.D. Thesis, CNAA,1980.

88. J. S. Garrow, in P. Bjorntorp et. al., Eds., *Recent Advances in Obesity Research*, Vol. 3, London, Libbey, 1981, p. 208.

7

Effects of Foods and Nutrients on Brain Neurotransmitters

RICHARD J. WURTMAN, M.D.

Laboratory of Neuroendocrine Regulation, Department of Nutrition and Food Science, Massachusetts Institute of Technology, Cambridge, Massachusetts

A large body of evidence affirms that the consumption of certain foods, or of pure nutrients extracted from those foods, can influence the rates at which some neurons synthesize and release their neurotransmitters. Moreover, the neurochemical effects of any meal bear a predictable relationship to its nutrient composition and to the individual's metabolic state at the time of its consumption (e.g., whether it is the initial meal of the day). Carbohydrate-rich or protein-rich meals change plasma amino acid levels so as to increase and decrease, respectively, brain tryptophan concentrations and serotonin synthesis; lecithin-rich foods elevate plasma and brain choline, thereby potentially accelerating acetylcholine production; and protein consumption (or the administration of tyrosine in pure form) can enhance catecholamine synthesis. Although it remains to be explained *why* the evolutionary process made the brain so susceptible to the vagaries of food choice, an understanding of *how* these nutrients affect brain composition may throw some light on normal and abnormal interactions between peripheral metabolism and brain function. It might also suggest new ways for treating disorders involving neurons that release the precursor-dependent neurotransmitters, and perhaps ways for improving sleep, mood, appetite control, and general performance among normal people. This chapter summarizes our understanding of precursor-neurotransmitter relationships, and describes how small variations in nutrition or metabolism can, by affecting precursor availability, influence the functioning of the nervous system.

103

FACTORS AFFECTING NEUROTRANSMISSION

The amount of information that a set of like neurons can transmit during a particular interval depends theoretically on three factors, the *number* of neurons in the set (or the number of synapses that these neurons make), the *average* frequency at which these neurons happen to be firing, and the average number of *neurotransmitter molecules* that the neuron releases each time it fires (1, 2). All of these factors are subject to change. The number of synapses might sometimes increase (if the brain is indeed "plastic," as some studies suggest); however the number of *neurons* clearly decreases, inexorably, with age. Any neuron's firing frequency will typically accelerate or decelerate many times during each day, increasing when it is bombarded with excitatory neurotransmitters released from other neurons, and decreasing in response to inhibitory transmitters. Evidence accumulated during the past decade has shown that the numbers of neurotransmitter molecules that some neurons release per firing can also vary over wide ranges, depending in part on the quantity of transmitters present at that instant in the presynaptic terminals. This quantity can, for serotonin, acetylcholine, and the catecholamines, increase or decrease when changes in plasma composition—as occur after eating—cause more or less of the transmitter's circulating precursor to be delivered to the neuron. In the case of serotonin, an increase in available precursor (tryptophan) apparently always will increase the transmitter's synthesis. For acetylcholine and the catecholamines, enhanced precursor availability will accelerate transmitter synthesis only with the brain's connivance, that is, only, in each neuron, when the brain causes that neuron to fire frequently—a relationship that imparts considerable physiologic specificity to the consequences of nutritional interventions affecting choline or tyrosine availability.

The general laws governing the relationships between the syntheses of these neurotransmitters and the plasma levels of their precursors can be summarized as follows:

1. The limiting step in the biosynthesis of the transmitter must be catalyzed by a low-affinity enzyme—tryptophan hydroxylase, choline acetyltransferase, or tyrosine hydroxylase—which, at normal substrate concentrations, is unsaturated with the precursor.

2. This enzyme must not be subject to significant end-product feedback control when the neuron containing it is firing frequently.

3. The amount of the enzyme's substrate (the neurotransmitter precursor) present within the neuron must depend on its concentration in the plasma, either because the nerve terminal is unable to make the precursor (e.g., tryptophan) and obtains it solely by *influx* from the plasma, or because, even though the neuron can synthesize the precursor (e.g., choline), it tends to lose it by efflux into the plasma at a rate that varies inversely with the precursor's plasma concentration.

4. A mechanism must exist which facilitates the precursor's passage from the bloodstream to the brain, and vice versa (i.e., a blood-brain barrier transport system); moreover the affinity of this mechanism for the circulating precursor must, like that of the rate-limiting enzyme, be relatively *low*. A physiologic increase in, for example, plasma tyrosine levels, must increase the transport system's saturation with tyrosine and must thereby facilitate tyrosine's entry into the brain.

As discussed below, a single transport mechanism, probably comprising a single system of macromolecules, mediates the facilitated diffusion of all of the large neutral amino acids (LNAA) across the blood-brain barrier (3). The K_m of this mechanism for LNAA, per se, is of the same order of magnitude as the total plasma LNAA concentration; hence each of the LNAAs competes with all of the others for uptake sites. As a consequence, the rate at which circulating tyrosine enters the brain depends both on plasma tyrosine levels and, inversely, on plasma levels of tryptophan, phenylalanine, leucine, isoleucine, and valine (and, to a lesser extent, on a few additional amino acids) (4, 5). The most important "competing LNAA," by virtue of their relatively high affinities for the carrier and their plasma concentrations, are the aromatic and branched-chain amino acids; hence brain tyrosine levels at any moment can be predicted by a plasma tyrosine ratio whose numerator is the concentration of tyrosine, and denominator the sum of the plasma concentrations of tryptophan, phenylalanine, and the branched-chain triad (5). Similar plasma ratios predict brain levels of tryptophan and other LNAA. The predictive power is slightly improved if more individual LNAAs are included in the denominator, and if corrections are made for differences in the affinities of individual LNAA for the transport carrier. In the case of circulating tryptophan, transport across the blood-brain barrier also is retarded to a very small extent by the amino acid's low-affinity, high-capacity binding to albumin. The power of the blood-brain barrier transport mechanisms to grab and hold circulating tryptophan is, generally, so much greater than that of circulating albumin that, for all practical purposes, no correction need usually be made in the plasma tryptophan ratio for that portion of circulating tryptophan which happens to be albumin-bound at the moment it enters brain capillaries (6).

No normal plasma constituents have been identified that significantly affect choline's flux from the brain to blood.

5.   Plasma levels of the precursors must, in fact, *change* under normal conditions. For example, choline levels must (and do) rise after choline is consumed (7) (as the free base or as a constituent of lecithin or sphingomyelin), and plasma LNAA (other than tryptophan) must be able to rise after protein is consumed, or to fall after carbohydrate consumption has elicited insulin secretion (8). (Plasma tryptophan increases only slightly after protein consumption, reflecting tryptophan's scarcity in protein, and is largely unaffected by insulin (9)).

NUTRIENT CONSUMPTION AND NEUROTRANSMITTER SYNTHESIS

Since plasma choline and LNAA levels are *not* regulated but rise or fall depending upon what is currently being digested and absorbed, food consumption assumes considerable importance as an at least potential determinant of brain function. Each meal produces, within minutes of its initiation, predictable changes in plasma choline (7) and LNAA (8) levels; minutes later, equally predictable changes are observed in brain neurotransmitters (10, 11). A meal rich in lecithin (or, for milk-consuming infants, sphingomyelin) rapidly elevates blood and brain choline levels; the lack of dietary choline for 12–24 hours causes a gradual fall in plasma choline (7, 12). A protein-poor meal, acting via insulin secretion, markedly reduces (by greater than 50%) plasma leucine, isoleucine, and valine levels without affecting plasma tryptophan (which is buffered by its loose binding to albumin (9, 13)). As a consequence the plasma tryptophan ratio increases, and brain serotonin quickly follows. This protein-poor meal also causes plasma tyrosine levels to fall, but not by so great a proportion as the branched-chain amino acids (12); hence the tyrosine ratio may increase slightly, causing a small acceleration in catecholamine synthesis and release within physiologically active neurons (14). Consumption of a high-protein meal causes a seemingly paradoxical fall in the tryptophan ratio (11), and a rise in the tyrosine ratio (5), followed by the anticipated changes in brain monoamine synthesis. The fall in the tryptophan ratio reflects tryptophan's scarcity in dietary protein (0.5–1.6% of total amino acids); even though plasma tryptophan *levels* do rise somewhat, this increase is far less than that of the competing LNAA. The rise in the tyrosine ratio after protein consumption reflects the fact that proteins contain *two* molecules that tend to elevate plasma tyrosine, that is, tyrosine itself and phenylalanine, much of which is converted to tyrosine in each pass through the portal circulation.

Serotonin-Releasing Neurons as Metabolic Sensors

Because serotonin-producing neurons exhibit characteristic inverse responses to the proportion of protein in each meal, they are able to function as "sensors" of food-induced changes in plasma composition. Throughout the range of plasma tryptophan ratios associated with eating protein-free to high-protein meals, serotonin neurons will produce (11) and release (15) more or less of their transmitter, thereby "informing" other brain neurons about the individual's metabolic state. That these other neurons actually use this information is shown by recent studies on the control of food selection. If rats (16, 17) or humans (18) are given a simultaneous choice of several diet mixtures containing different proportions of carbohydrate and protein, it is observed that treatments (i.e., tryptophan, fenfluramine, fluoxetine, MK-212) that enhance serotoninergic transmission cause subjects to choose to diminish the proportion of mealtime calories represented by carbohydrates, and increase that of protein. One can thus hypothesize that one reason that evolution "allowed" serotonin neurons to be open-loop with respect to plasma composition was so that these neurons could serve as "sensors," in a behavioral feedback loop designed to keep these proportions within desired ranges. Perhaps impairments in this hypothetical loop predispose to carbohydrate craving with or without resulting obesity. Carbohydrate-induced (or tryptophan-induced) increases in serotonin synthesis also facilitate some cyclic biologic processes (like sleep onset and growth hormone secretion), and tend to raise the individual's threshold for perceiving pain and various exteroceptive stimuli. The most effective nutrient mixture for enhancing brain serotonin synthesis would include a low dose of tryptophan (i.e., not so high as to suppress brain uptake of tyrosine and other LNAA), mixed with an amount of carbohydrate (19) sufficient to cause insulin secretion.

TYROSINE AND THE SYNTHESIS AND RELEASE OF CATECHOLAMINES

Administration of tryptophan leads to rapid elevations in brain serotonin (11); in contrast, tyrosine administration has little effect on brain catecholamine levels. This apparently negative relationship initially led investigators to assume that catecholamine synthesis was not under significant precursor control. It was not until studies using decarboxylase inhibitors showed that the rate at which brain catechols are formed does vary with brain tyrosine levels (4) that this earlier view was challenged. From a position of hindsight, it is possible to understand why precursor control of catecholamine synthesis was so late in being recognized. The fact that brain dopamine or norepinephrine levels do not change appreciably in the hour or two after tyrosine administration may reflect the relatively slow turnover of these transmitters (compared with that of serotonin) and the heterogeneity of their storage compartments. It is possible that even a doubling in the synthesis of the most important norepinephrine pool would not cause a detectable rise in brain norepinephrine levels until many hours had passed (because other, larger pools turn over so slowly). It is also possible that tyrosine-induced changes in transmitter levels do exist within particular brain regions, but are not detectable in large brain samples. In any case, abundant evidence has since been obtained that tyrosine levels can influence not only the synthesis of brain catecholamines, but also their rates of *release* (as reflected by brain levels of the dopamine metabolites DOPAC and HVA and the norepinephrine metabolite MOPEG-SO$_4$).

The extent to which catecholaminergic neurons are affected by tyrosine levels seems to depend on their firing frequencies. Dopamine release from nigrostriatal neurons under resting conditions is unaffected by even major changes in tyrosine levels, but is markedly enhanced following treatment with haloperidol (20) or reserpine (which block dopamine receptors and dopamine storage, respectively), or partial lesioning of the nigrostriatal tract (21) (which accelerates the firing of the surviving neurons). Norepinephrine release is enhanced slightly in brains of otherwise untreated animals when brain tyrosine levels have been elevated, but this effect is potentiated when noradrenergic neurons are caused to fire more rapidly than normal (e.g., in hypertensive rats (22), or among animals placed in a cold environment). A relationship between neuronal firing rates and precursor dependence also characterizes cholinergic neurons. For example, the choline concentration in the medium has little effect on the *spontaneous* release of acetylcholine from motor neurons innervating the rat diaphragm, but markedly augments the acetylcholine release caused by stimulating the phrenic nerve electrically (23). (The particular mechanism that couples neuronal firing rate to tyrosine dependence apparently involves phosphorylation of the tyrosine hydroxylase enzyme protein, which increases the enzyme's affinity for its cofactor, tetrahydrobiopterin, causing it to become more limited by tyrosine. The mechanism coupling the choline dependence of cholinergic neurons to their firing frequency awaits discovery.)

Circulating tyrosine levels can effectively be elevated by giving people large oral doses of the amino acid (24, 25). Concurrent protein consumption dampens the rise in the plasma tyrosine ratio, but this can be overcome by increasing the dose. Giving tyrosine with an appropriate quantity of carbohydrate (to elicit insulin secretion and diminish plasma levels of the branched-chain amino acids) markedly enhances its effect on brain tyrosine levels in the rat (26).

WHEN MIGHT NEUROTRANSMITTER SYNTHESIS AFFECT NEUROTRANSMITTER RELEASE?

Under what conditions might a change in neurotransmitter *synthesis*, caused by giving its precursor, be expected to modify the amount of transmitter *released* each time the neuron fires? A decade ago one might have answered "never," basing one's conclusions on the likelihood that the transmitter molecules released into synapses came from synaptic vesicles, and that the average number of molecules present in each vesicle was fairly constant. At present it no longer is certain that the transmitter released into synapses *when neurons fire* actually comes from vesicles. Moreover, the increases in brain levels of monoamine metabolites (HVA, MOPEG-SO$_4$, 5-HIAA) after tyrosine or tryptophan administration render moot arguments based on where in the neuron "releasable" neurotransmitter molecules happen to be stored. Thus the question deserves an answer.

It seems clear that the central nervous system could easily buffer whatever effects tyrosine or choline administration might have on *neurotransmission,* simply by diminishing neuronal firing rates. If, for example, each brain cholinergic neuron released twice as much acetylcholine per firing as a result of choline administration, the brain could keep this change from seriously affecting neurotransmission by reducing firing rates by half. There are three conditions under which we might expect such modulation *not* to occur:

1. If the neurons in question are "designed" to function as sensors, coupling their output signal (neurotransmitter release per unit time) to the level of something being sensed (for example, the plasma tryptophan ratio, postprandially). In this circumstance, their design would include the absence of multisynaptic feedback loops for suppressing their firing rates when transmitter release per firing increases.

2. If neurotransmitter release is not controlled by multisynaptic feedback loops (e.g., release from peripheral autonomic or motor neurons, or adrenal medulla). Thus, for example, choline administration causes major and prolonged increases in preganglionic neurotransmission, as reflected by epinephrine release from the adrenal medulla (27) and tyrosine hydroxylase induction in the medulla (28) and in sympathetic ganglia; tyrosine administration also causes prolonged increases in human urinary norepinephrine and epinephrine levels (29).

3. If the neurons are "sick" and are unable to release as much transmitters as the brain would "like" (e.g., because they are too few in number, as in Alzheimer's disease, or Parkinson's disease, or are physiologically impaired, as in tardive dyskinesia), or if they are tonically activated because of some overriding physiologic need (e.g., brainstem noradrenergic neurons in hypertension (22) or sympathoadrenal cells in shock) (30).

USE OF NEUROTRANSMITTER PRECURSORS TO TREAT DISORDERS INVOLVING NEURONS

This third situation underlies the current interest in therapeutic uses of neurotransmitter precursors. It seems likely that, if a particular precursor-dependent transmitter (e.g., dopamine) is utilized by a number of different brain tracts, and if but one of the tracts is "sick," or diminished by age, then its function may be selectively restored by giving tyrosine, without causing excessive dopaminergic tone in the other, "healthy," dopaminergic tracts. Available clinical and experimental evidence, though meager, tends to support this expectation. For example, tyrosine administration increases hypothalamic dopamine synthesis and thereby reduces pituitary prolactin secretion in *hyperprolactenemia*, but not where prolactin levels are normal (31). Its administration to patients with mild Parkinson's disease can diminish their clinical signs without causing the signs of dopaminergic hyperactivity seen with dopaminergic agonists (nausea, hallucinations, psychosis) (32). Tyrosine rapidly increases brainstem MOPEG-SO$_4$ levels and lowers blood pressure in hypertensive animals, but has relatively little effect on either index in normotensives (22). Choline (or lecithin) and physostigmine share an ability to ameliorate the signs of tardive dyskinesia (33), but precursor administration fails to produce the marked side effects, characteristic of generalized cholinergic activation, seen with physostigmine. It will be fortunate indeed if future studies bear out the apparent ability of neurotransmitter precursor molecules to *target* their sites of action to those synapses at which more of their transmitter products happen to be needed. A major group of beneficiaries will be the aged. One might foresee the production of tonics for the aged, providing all of the relevant neurotransmitter precursors, the consumption of which would enable individual brain neurons to choose whether they wished to have their transmission properties amplified.

REFERENCES

1. R. J. Wurtman, *Scientific American*, **246**, 42 (1982).
2. R. J. Wurtman, F. Hefti, and E. Melamed, *Pharm. Rev.*, **32**, 315 (1981).
3. W. M. Pardridge, *Nutrition and the Brain*, Vol. 1, New York, Raven, 1977, pp. 141-204.
4. R. J. Wurtman, F. Larin, S. Mostafapour, and J. D. Fernstrom, *Science, 195*, 183 (1974).

5.   J. D. Fernstrom and D. V. Faller, *J. Neurochem.*, **25**, 825 (1978).

6.   R. J. Wurtman and W. M. Pardridge, *J. Neural. Transm.*, Suppl. **15**, 227 (1979).

7.   M. H. Hirsch, J. H. Growdon and R. J. Wurtman, *Metabolism*, **27**, 952 (1978).

8.   R. J. Wurtman, C. M. Rose, C. Chou, and F. Larin, New Engl. J. Med., **279**, 171 (1968).

9.   J. D. Fernstrom, R. J. Wurtman, B. Hammarstrom-Wiklund, W. M. Rand, H. N Munro, and C. S. Davidson, *Am. J. Clin. Nutr.*, **32**, 1923 (1979).

10.   E. L. Cohen and R. J. Wurtman, *Science*, **191**, 651 (1976).

11.   J. D. Fernstrom and R. J. Wurtman, *Science*, **178**, 414 (1972).

12.   R. J. Wurtman, M. J. Hirsch, and J. H. Growdon, *Lancet*, **2**, 68 (1977).

13.   R. J. Wurtman, *Mammalian Protein Metabolism*, Vol. IV, New York, Academic, 1970, pp. 445-480.

14.   C. J. Gibson and R. J. Wurtman, *Life Sci.*, **22**, 1399 (1978).

15.   J. L. Colmenares, R. J. Wurtman, and J. D. Fernstrom, *J. Neurochem.*, **25**, 825 (1975).

16.   J. J. Wurtman and R. J. Wurtman, *Science*, **198**, 1178 (1977).

17.   J. J. Wurtman and R. J. Wurtman, *Life Sci.*, **24**, 895 (1979).

18.   J. J. Wurtman, R. J. Wurtman, J. H. Growdon, P. Henry, A. Lipscomb, and S. H. Zeisel, *Int. J. Eating Disorders*, **1**, 2 (1981).

19.   R. Martin-Du Pan, C. Mauron, B. Glaeser, and R. J. Wurtman, *Metabolism*, **31**, 937 (1982).

20.   M. C. Scally, I. H. Ulus, and R. J. Wurtman, *J. Neural. Transm.*, **41**, 1 (1977).

21.   F. Hefti, E. Melamed, and R. J. Wurtman, *Brain Res.*, **195**, 123 (1980).

22.   A. F. Sved, J. D. Fernstrom, and R. J. Wurtman, *Proc. Natl. Acad Sci.*, USA, **76**, 3511 (1979).

23.   G. G. Bierkamper and A. M. Goldberg, In A. Barbeau, J. H. Growdon, and R. J. Wurtman, Eds., *Choline and Lecithin in Brain Disorders, Nutrition and the Brain*, Vol. 5, New York, Raven, 1979, pp. 252-253.

24.   B. Glaeser, E. Melamed, J. H. Growdon, and R. J. Wurtman, *Life Sci.*, **24**, 265 (1979).

25.   E. Melamed, B. Glaeser, J. H. Growdon, and R. J. Wurtman, *Life Sci.* (in press).

26.   C. Mauron and R. J. Wurtman, *J. Neural. Transm.* (in press).

27.   M. C. Scally, I. H. Ulus, and R. J. Wurtman, *J. Neural. Transm.*, **43**, 103 (1978).

28.   I. H. Ulus, M. C. Scally, and R. J. Wurtman, *J. Pharmacol. Exp. Ther.*, **204**, 676 (1978).

29.   J. Agharanya, R. Alonso, and R. J. Wurtman, *Am J. Clin. Nutr.*, **34**, 82 (1981).

30.   L. A. Conlay, T. J. Maher, and R. J. Wurtman, *Science*, **212**, 559 (1981).

31.   A. F. Sved, J. D. Fernstrom, and R. J. Wurtman, *Life Sci.*, **25**, 1293 (1979).

32.   J. H. Growdon, E. Melamed, M. Logue, F. Hefti, and R. J. Wurtman, *Life Sci.*, **30**, 827 (1982).

33.   A Barbeau, J. H. Growdon and R. J. Wurtman, *Choline and Lecithin in Brain Disorders, Nutrition and the Brain*, Vol. V, New York, Raven, 1979.

8

The Assessment of the Functional Consequences of Malnutrition

DAVID McR. RUSSELL, MBBS, FRACP, and
KHURSHEED N. JEEJEEBHOY, MBBS, Ph.D.,
FRCP(C)

Department of Medicine, University of Toronto, Toronto General Hospital, Toronto, Ontario, Canada

The diagnosis of protein-calorie malnutrition is often based on objective measurements of nutritional status, including assessment of body composition (including anthropometric evaluation, total body nitrogen (TBN), and total body potassium (TBK)), creatinine-height index, nitrogen balance, hepatic secretory proteins, and the degree of immunocompetence. Although it is easy to characterize the severely malnourished patient by using these objective measurements, the exact recognition of early and subtle malnutrition is not as simple. Since this recognition and knowledge of the effects of early malnutrition are both important in defining the need for nutritional support, several investigators have related a variety of parameters of body compositions and biochemistry to the risks of infection, postoperative complications, and death (1–6). Unfortunately, there has been no consistent relationship between these parameters of nutritional assessment and prognosis.

In part, this is because the prognosis of a patient hinges not only on the nutritional status, but also on the nature of the illness and treatment, and the presence of sepsis. However, another reason for this descrepancy may be that the functional effects of malnutrition are often

Supported in part by the Ontario Ministry of Health (Grant PR 228), the Medical Research Council of Canada (Grant MA-7923), and various sponsors.

not manifested by significant changes in traditional measurements of body composition. Hence morbidity and mortality may correlate better with the deleterious effects of malnutrition on organ function than with the changes in body composition. In this chapter we will consider the effects of malnutrition on three separate and vital organ functions, namely (1) hepatic secretory protein function, (2) immunocompetence, and (3) skeletal muscle function.

HEPATIC SECRETORY PROTEINS

A variety of proteins, including prealbumin, albumin, transferrin, ceruloplasmin, and retinol-binding protein, are synthesized by the liver and secreted into the plasma. Albumin is the most abundant of these proteins, and the human serum contains 35 to 45 g per liter. In the hepatocyte, it is not native albumin that is formed but a precursor known as prealbumin, which differs from native albumin by 24 additional amino acid residues (7). It takes 25 to 30 minutes for a molecule of albumin to be synthesized by the polysomes and secreted into the plasma (8). Albumin is not stored in the hepatocyte, but is continuously secreted into the plasma at an estimated rate of 17 g per day, and turned over with a half-life of approximately 21 days (8). Nutrient supply is critical for the maintenance of the polysomal aggregation required for optimal protein synthesis, and it has been clearly established that total hepatic protein and RNA levels decline during fasting (7,9). Hence in conditions of deficient input, it might be expected that the plasma concentration of albumin and other plasma proteins secreted by the liver, namely transferrin and retinol-binding protein, would decline. The rate of decline in the serum levels of any of these proteins due to reduced synthesis is proportional to the rate of turnover (i.e., inversely proportional to half-life).

While a low serum albumin may indicate depletion of visceral protein, because of its long half-life, changes in synthesis will not alter circulating levels rapidly. Several clinical studies have demonstrated this delayed response, showing that serum albumin does not respond to short-term changes in protein and energy intake, compared with prealbumin and retinol-binding protein (10,11). The levels of these latter two proteins in turn changed more rapidly in response to both dietary restriction and refeeding.

One of the intrinsic difficulties in using the plasma concentration of these hepatic secretory proteins in the assessment of nutritional status is the problem of separating the effects of actual nutrient deprivation from those of the disease process. The plasma level of these proteins critically depends on liver function. Altered liver function due to septicemia and underlying liver disease, and excessive protein losses (e.g., protein-losing enteropathy) may account for low serum albumin levels even when nutrients are available in sufficient quantities (12,13). Hence the conclusion that nutrient deficiency per se can be adequately assessed by measuring plasma protein levels is probably not justified.

IMMUNODEFICIENCY

Malnutrition is the commonest cause of secondary immunodeficiency. This alteration in immune function affects almost all facets of host resistance and as a result, infection is one of the most frequent complications of undernutrition. Cell-mediated immune response is affected earlier and more severely by undernutrition. In malnutrition it has been demonstrated that the proportion and absolute numbers of T cells are decreased (14), the function of T helper cells is impaired, and T-cell differentiation may be retarded because of reduction in thymic inductive hormones (15).

In addition to impaired cell-mediated immunity, the complement system, opsonic function of plasma, and polymorphonuclear cell function may also be altered in severe malnutrition. Recently the phagocytic role of a high molecular weight glycoprotein, fibronectin, has been extensively studied. Fibronectin is found in blood and tissue fluid as well as in association with basement membranes, connective tissue, and the extracellular matrix of many cells (16–19). The site of synthesis of the opsonically active plasma fibronectin remains to be delineated. In tissue culture, fibronectin is actively produced by vascular endothelial cells, fibroblasts and hepatocytes, and some macrophages (16,18,19). Plasma fibronectin is known to aid phagocytic function of macrophages such as the Kupffer cell. Multiple organ failure in the septic patient may be related to Kupffer cell dysfunction mediated by plasma opsonic fibronectin deficiency (20). Plasma fibronectin deficiency has also been noted in patients with major burn injury (21) and during starvation in rats (20). Deficiency of plasma opsonic fibronectin in septic injured patients can be reversed by intravenous infusion of fibronectin-rich fresh plasma cryoprecipitate (22). However, this form of therapy is still experimental. The levels of opsonic fibronectin are sensitive to disturbed nutrition and thus host defense mechanisms may be impaired in malnutrition by fibronectin deficiency.

Severe undernutrition also alters serum immunoglobulins. Serum immunoglobulin G (IgG) concentration is usually elevated (23), although rarely it may be low, particularly in low birth weight marasmic infants (24). Secretory immunoglobulin A (IgA) and mucosal antibody responses to viral antigens are usually reduced. This may be due to a reduction in IgA-producing plasma cells, reduced synthesis of secretory component, or decreased T-cell function (25).

Selected nutrient deficiencies can also alter immune function. Zinc deficiency is associated with lymphoid atrophy and decreased delayed cutaneous hypersensitivity (26). Iron and magnesium deficiency can impair in vitro immune function testing and are associated with an increased incidence of certain infections (27). Deficiencies of pyridoxine, folic acid, vitamin A, and vitamin E may result in impaired cell-mediated immunity and reduced antibody responses (28).

The most common form of in vivo testing of immunocompetence in hospitalized patients is delayed cutaneous hypersensitivity (DCH) to known recall antigens. The common antigens tested by intradermal injection include mumps, candida, streptokinase-streptodornase, purified protein derivative (PPD), dinitrochlorobenzene (DNCB), and, in pediatrics, diphtheria toxoid. At least three antigens are injected intradermally on the forearm and read at 24 and 48 hours. Greater than 10 mm of induration is considered positive, and a patient is considered anergic if he does not react to any of the three antigens. Meakins (2) showed that increased postoperative infection and decreased survival were seen in patients with absent DCH (1). They considered the cause of such anergy to be malnutrition. However, it is well known that a number of factors other than undernutrition can suppress DCH (29). The following factors must be taken into account before attributing abnormalities of skin test response to malnutrition alone:

1. *Infections.* Sepsis due to viral (30,31), bacterial (32), and granulomatous infections (33) can suppress normal DCH. Therefore, it is not surprising that it was subsequently shown that simply draining the site of infection could reverse anergy (34).

2. *Metabolic Disorders.* Uremia (35,36), cirrhosis (37,38), hepatitis (39,40), inflammatory bowel diseases (41–43), and sarcoidosis (44–46) are known to suppress normal DCH. It appears that trauma alone in the absence of malnutrition can produce anergy (47), and perhaps burns (48) and hemorrhage (49,50) alone can alter DCH.

3. *Malignant Disease* Anergy or depressed DCH has been noted in patients with solid tumors (30). Chemotherapy (51) and radiotherapy (52–54) are also known to impair DCH.

4. *Drugs.* Many commonly used drugs affect DCH, including steroids (55,56), immunosuppressents (57), cimetidine (58–60), coumadin (61), and perhaps aspirin (62).

5. *Surgery and Anesthesia.* General anesthesia alone, even in the absence of surgery, can depress immune function and change DCH (63).

Clearly the abnormalities in DCH in the hospitalized patient are nonspecific and do not necessarily reflect a state of nutrient deficiency. Hence proof that the malnutrition associated with absent DCH is a major cause of increased morbidity or mortality is equivocal. It may be that stress with elevated steroid levels, present in many diseases and in malnutrition, is a common pathway to depressed skin test response.

SKELETAL MUSCLE FUNCTION

Wasting of muscle is an obvious effect of severe malnutrition, and has led to the use of anthropometric measurements, including limb muscle circumference, to assess malnutrition. Based on the assumption that a positive nitrogen balance indicates muscle anabolism, a positive nitrogen balance has been used as an index of the beneficial effects of nutritional support. In animal experiments (with growing rats) and in young children, nitrogen retention and growth are obvious effects of optimum nutritional intake. This observation has been applied to malnourished adult humans (nongrowing) who have been considered potentially able to "regrow" the lost tissue.

Although it is true that patients receiving long-term home total parenteral nutrition (TPN) gain body weight and nitrogen over many months and years of observation, this process is not seen in shorter and intermediate term nutritional intervention given in hospital (64). Thus, despite adequate intake of nitrogen and calories, little or no increase in total body nitrogen was seen in a variety of patients receiving TPN in hospital over several weeks. If, however, the nitrogen intake is markedly increased, then some gain in nitrogen is observed (65). In contrast to the absent or very modest gain in nitrogen, nutritional support does appear to improve outcome in the form of reduced complications and mortality after a period of support so short that body composition is hardly altered. For example, it has been shown that amino acids and amino acids plus calories both resulted in equivalent sparing of body nitrogen, but the latter was associated with quicker wound healing and fewer complications (66). It has also been shown that patients with reduced plasma protein levels and absent DCH had increased postoperative morbidity improved by a 7-day course of preoperative nutritional support (5). However, these same investigators noted that improvement was not associated with a change or improvement in the very indices used to predict the presence of malnutrition (Prognostic Nutritional Index). Other investigators have demonstrated that a 10-day period of preoperative nutritional support altered morbidity and mortality following surgery in patients with gastrointestinal carcinoma (6).

Thus the outcome and body composition data suggest that the reversal of the adverse effects of malnutrition was not based on improvement of the traditional parameters of nutrition, such as gain in body nitrogen or a demonstrated increase in muscle mass or in plasma proteins. Concordant with this discrepancy is the observation that global clinical assessment is at least equivalent to, and in some respects better than, individual objective traditional measurements of nutritional status in predicting outcome (67).

On the basis of the foregoing evidence, there are grounds for suspecting that functional abnormalities in adult (nongrowing) humans may not be the result of simple loss of lean tissue and may disappear before any such lean tissue is regained.

To investigate this area we have done a series of three studies using objective measurements of muscle function in relation to nutritional deprivation and refeeding in humans and in an animal model.

Muscle Function Tests

We examined a function that could be measured objectively, namely, the muscle contraction-relaxation characteristics (in contrast to pure force) and endurance. Muscle function was chosen because the reduced protein stores and catabolism that occur in malnutrition seemed likely to alter muscle contractility, relaxation rate, and endurance at an early stage of the process. Muscle function is of vital importance because changes in the ability to contract and relax quickly, and reduced endurance, may alter respiratory function and lead to respiratory failure in critically ill patients.

It has been shown consistently that the ratio of body potassium to sodium is altered in malnutrition (68,69). These changes could alter the intracellular electrolyte content and thus the responsiveness of muscle, and hence muscle function could be altered before these changes could be detected by whole body measurements. During a period of deficient nutrient intake such changes in muscle function could precede detectable changes in structure or composition. Through an objective study of muscle function in response to deficient nutrient intake, we could, in theory, define at what point functional impairment commences.

Human studies.   There are problems in testing for muscle strength and fatigue. The straightforward approach would be to exercise the patient, measuring performance on a treadmill or bicycle. Obviously this is not possible with seriously ill patients, and furthermore the result depends on previous training and motivation. More important, during the initial phases of contraction, the nerve impulses are rapid. As high frequency fatigue sets in, the rate of impulse slows. Thus voluntary contraction has an inbuilt reserve mechanism that does not allow the demonstration of early abnormality. To avoid these obstacles it was necessary to use a more controlled objective method of stimulating the muscle which does not depend on voluntary effort by the patient. The method we chose involves electrical stimulation of the ulnar nerve at the wrist and measurement of the contraction characteristics of the adductor pollicis muscle.

The techniques for objective muscle testing were originally described by Merton (70) and more recently have been modified by Edwards (71,72). It has also been shown that the measurements of muscle function as described by Merton and Edwards will give the same results when diverse muscles, such as the adductor pollicis, quadriceps, sternomastoid, and diaphragm, are tested (73). The similarity of the results from diverse muscles allows us to consider the function of the adductor pollicis representative of muscle function as a whole. In preliminary studies we have confirmed that the diaphragmatic changes in malnutrition mirror those in the adductor pollicis. Thus the studies to be described may be representative of a vital muscle mass such as the diaphragm. We studied the function of the adductor pollicis muscle in the right hand by stimulating the ulnar nerve at the wrist with an electrical unidirectional square wave impulse of 75–100 microsecond duration. The stimulus was of a supramaximal voltage (range 80–120 V) and at frequencies increasing from 10 to 100 Hz. Simultaneous EMG records documented constant supramaximal nerve stimulation.

This technique involved minor discomfort but not pain. When the motor nerve to a muscle is stimulated at a voltage at least 20% greater than that needed to achieve a maximum mechanical or electrical response (supramaximal nerve stimulation) all muscle fibers are made to contract. The force generated depends on the frequency of stimulation and whether the muscle is fresh or fatigued. Absolute forces vary among individuals, depending on body size and muscular training. However, the force obtained at different stimulation frequencies expressed as a percentage of the maximal force produced by electrical stimulation (force-frequency curve) is reproducible and comparable among individuals. Electrical stimulation of the ulnar nerve at 10, 20, 30, 50, and 100 Hz with 15–30 second intervals between the stimuli has been performed (Figure 8-1). This procedure has been repeated to test the reproducibility. The effects of posttetanic potentiation have been standardized by a fixed order of testing. In normal healthy subjects at low frequency stimulation, the muscle responds as single twitches that generate a small percentage of the maximum force. As the stimulus frequency increases the twitches start to fuse and the force increases. Above 20 Hz the muscle is tetanized, and above 50 Hz the force is equal to the maximum voluntary force. The shape of this frequency curve is the same for different muscles and the same in all normal individuals. In the malnourished patient, tetany occurs at a lower stimulation frequency with potentiation of the muscle force. There is also a loss of force at high frequency stimulation, so that the force at 10 Hz expressed as a percentage of the force at 100 Hz (F_{10}/F_{max}) is increased.

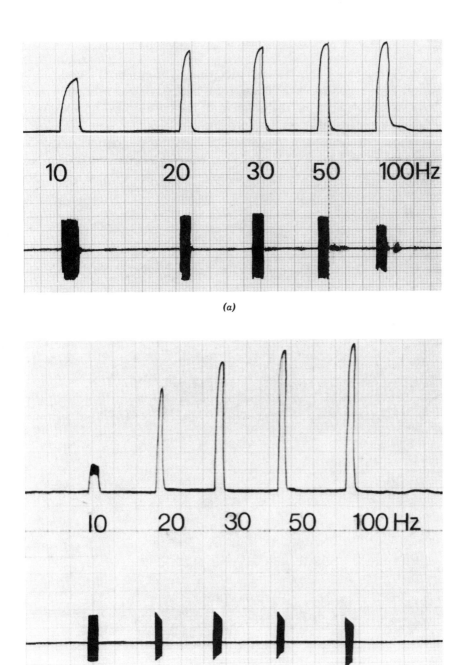

Figure 8-1. The force of contraction with electrical stimulation at 10, 20, 30, 50, and 100 Hz. A typical malnourished patient (Figure 8-1a) shows an increased force at 10 Hz (expressed as a per cent of the force at 100 Hz) compared with a normal subject. In Figure 8-1b the lower tracing in each graph shows the surface EMG, demonstrating constant nerve stimulation.

Muscle relaxation rate has been determined after a brief tetanic stimulation (1–2 seconds) at 30 Hz (Figure 8-2). Maximal relaxation rate (MRR) is calculated from the gradient of the initial phase of relaxation (74), and is expressed as percent force lost per 10 milliseconds. Although relaxation rate from voluntary isometric quadriceps contractions does increase with the force of contraction, electrically stimulated contractions producing increasing forces do not significantly change the MRR. Malnutrition results in significant slowing of the MRR of the adductor pollicis.

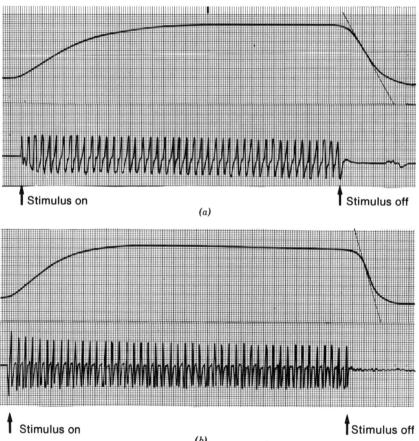

Figure 8-2. The force of contraction (and EMG recording) after a brief tetanic stimulation at 30 Hz in a typical malnourished patient (Figure 8-2a) and a normal subject (Figure 8-2b). The maximal relaxation rate is calculated from the gradient of the initial phase of relaxation (dotted line), and is slower in the malnourished patient.

Endurance was tested with continuous electrical stimulation at 20 Hz for 30 seconds duration, and the percent force loss/30 seconds was noted (Figure 8-3). Malnutrition resulted in significant muscle fatigue during prolonged stimulation.

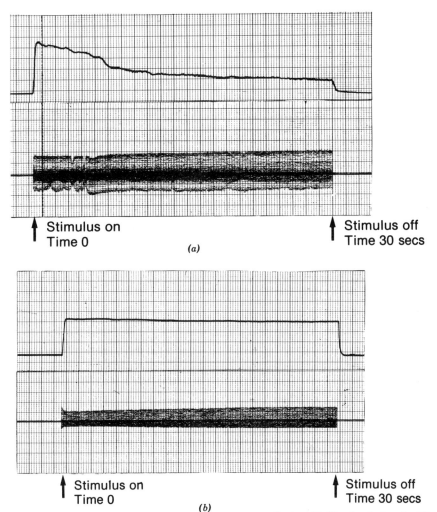

↑ Stimulus on
  Time 0

(a)

↑ Stimulus off
  Time 30 secs

↑ Stimulus on
  Time 0

(b)

↑ Stimulus off
  Time 30 secs

Figure 8-3.   The force of contraction (and EMG recording) at 20 Hz stimulation for 30 seconds, in a typical malnourished patient (Figure 8-3a) and a normal subject (Figure 8-3b). There is significant muscle fatigue in the malnourished patient compared with the normal subject.

Animal studies.   Barbiturate-anesthetized 8-week-old male Wistar rats had the gastrocnemius muscle freed with an intact blood supply and its nerve supply isolated. The body and hind limbs of the animal were immersed in modified Liley's solution kept at 37°C. The same measurements were made as in the human, but at frequencies from 0.5 to 200 Hz, noting the effects of stimulating the sciatic nerve on the contraction characteristics of the gastrocnemius muscle. Simultaneously biopsies were taken from the contralateral gastrocnemius and soleus muscles.

Effect of Malnutrition and Nutritional Support on Skeletal Muscle Function

Specific abnormalities in muscle function were observed in 10 patients with a variety of gastrointestinal disorders (75). All patients had clinical and biochemical features of severe nutritional depletion. Three discrete abnormalities of muscle function were noted: (1) altered force-frequency pattern with an increased force at 10 Hz stimulation expressed as a percent of the maximal force (increased F_{10}/F_{max}), (2) slower maximal relaxation rate, and (3) increased muscle fatigability. To assess the sensitivity of this technique of muscle function testing, six morbidly obese subjects were studied initially and after 2 weeks of a 400 kcal/day diet, again after an additional 2 weeks of fasting, and finally after 2 weeks of refeeding (76). Significant changes in muscle contraction-relaxation characteristics were noted after the 2 weeks of hypcaloric dieting, and even more profound changes of decreased MRR and increased muscle fatigability were noted after the 2 weeks of fasting. Oral refeeding resulted in restoration of all muscle function parameters to normal within 2 weeks (Figures 8-4–8-6).

To assess whether prolonged reduced nutrient input specifically alters skeletal muscle function, we also studied six patients with primary anorexia nervosa at a time of severe nutritional depletion, and then sequentially during strictly supervised oral refeeding (77). This study confirmed that pure protein-calorie malnutrition was associated with profound changes in muscle function, that after 4 weeks of oral refeeding muscle endurance and maximal relaxation rate were normal, and that by 8 weeks of refeeding all parameters were normal (Figures 8-7–8-9).

To confirm that the observations in humans were clearly related to nutritional deprivation, we studied the same functional parameters, together with metabolic analyses of muscle biopsies, in rats acutely deprived of nutrients or chronically underfed (as compared with pair-fed

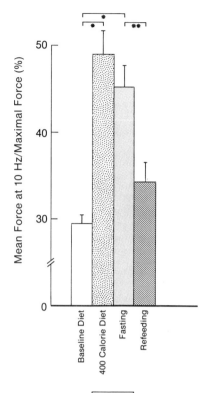

Figure 8-4. The changes in muscle force in six morbidly obese subjects while on a baseline diet (2500 kcal/day), and after 2 weeks of hypocaloric dieting (400 kcal/day), a further 2 weeks of fasting, and finally after 2 weeks of refeeding (approx. 1000 kcal/day). The bar graphs represent the mean ± SEM force at 10 Hz stimulation (expressed as a percentage of the maximal force). The brackets above the bar graphs indicate the significant changes during the study. $*p < 0.01$, $**p < 0.02$.

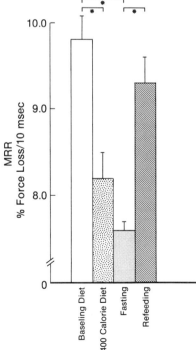

Figure 8-5. The changes in muscle maximal relaxation rate (MRR) in the same six morbidly obese subjects during the regimen noted in Figure 8-4. The bar graphs represent the mean ± SEM MRR. The brackets above the bar graphs indicate the significant changes during the study. $*p < 0.01$.

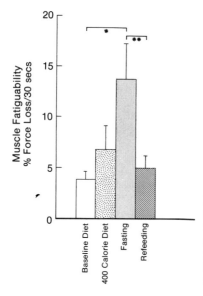

Figure 8-6. The changes in muscle fatigability in the same six morbidly obese subjects during the regimen noted in Figure 8-4. The bar graphs represent the mean ± SEM muscle fatigability. The brackets above the bar graphs indicate the significant changes during the study. *p < 0.01, **p < 0.05.

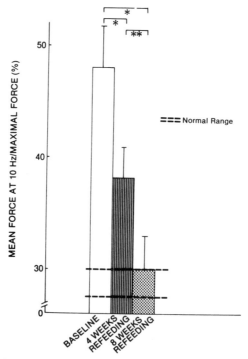

Figure 8-7. The changes in muscle force in six severely nutritionally depleted patients with anorexia nervosa at baseline and after 4 weeks and then 8 weeks of oral refeeding. The bar graphs represent the mean ± SEM force at 10Hz stimulation (expressed as a percentage of the maximal force). The brackets above the graphs indicate the significant changes during refeeding. *$p < 0.025$ **$p < 0.05$. The dotted lines represent the previously reported normal range (75). The F_{10}/F_{max} was restored to normal within 8 weeks of refeeding.

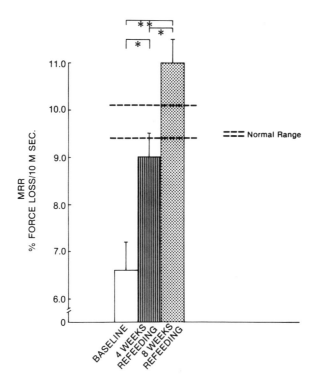

Figure 8-8.   The changes in muscle maximal relaxation rate (MRR) in the same six severely nutritionally depleted patients during the same regimen as in Figure 8-7. The bar
graphs represent the mean ± SEM MRR. The brackets above the graphs indicate the significant changes during refeeding. *$p < 0.05$ **$p < 0.001$. The dotted lines represent the
previously reported normal range (75). The MRR was restored to normal within 4 weeks
of refeeding.

animals). This animal model produced similar changes in skeletal function assessed by stimulating the sciatic nerve and measuring the function
of the gastrocnemius muscle. It also allowed us to analyze muscle composition in order to understand better the mechanisms responsible for
changes in muscle function in malnutrition.

Correlation of Objective Measurements of Body Composition and Muscle Function

The starved obese human did not lose significant amounts of TBK or
TBN, nor was there a significant change in creatinine-height index at a
time when abnormalities of muscle function were obvious (76). Con-

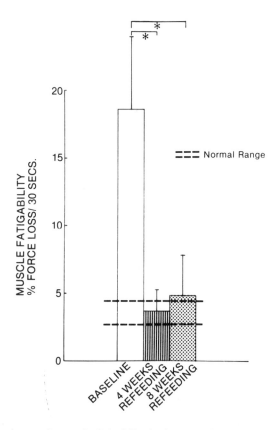

Figure 8-9. The changes in muscle fatigability in the same six severely nutritionally depleted patients during the same regimen as in Figure 8-7. The bar graphs represent the mean ± SEM muscle fatigability. The brackets above the bar graphs indicate the significant changes during refeeding. *$p < 0.05$. The dotted lines represent the previously reported normal range (75). Muscle fatigability returned rapidly to normal during refeeding.

versely, during refeeding these subjects rapidly lost muscle fatigability and had normal contraction-relaxation characteristics at a time when there was no significant increase in lean body components or in body weight.

In the anorexic patients, gross muscle fatigue and abnormal function were present when they were first seen (77). However, it was noted that these patients had normal plasma proteins at that time (Table 8-1). Ini-

Table 8.1 Changes in Standard Parameters of Nutritional Assessment During Oral Refeeding of Patients with Anorexia Nervosa

	Total Body Weight (kg)	Lean Body Weight (kg)	Body Fat (%)	Serum Albumin (g/dl)	Serum Transferrin (µg/dl)	Creatinine Height Index (%)	Lymphocyte Count (mm³)	DCH (No. anergic patients)
A. Baseline	39.0 ± 3.9	33.5 ± 3.2	14.0 ± 0.5	4.0 ± 0.1	170 ± 44	49.7 ± 7.4	1845 ± 252	5/6
B. Two weeks refeeding	41.1 ± 3.6	34.9 ± 3.1	15.0 ± 0.7	4.2 ± 0.4	228 ± 45	57.7 ± 6.1	1747 ± 220	—
C. Four weeks refeeding	43.4 ± 3.7	36.6 ± 3.1	15.7 ± 0.8	4.4 ± 0.3	215 ± 38	64.9 ± 3.4	2013 ± 315	3/6
D. Six weeks refeeding	44.8 ± 3.8	37.7 ± 2.9	16.8 ± 0.8	4.5 ± 0.3	243 ± 41	63.4 ± 4.1	1727 ± 262	—
E. Eight weeks refeeding	46.5 ± 4.4	38.6 ± 3.4	17.1 ± 1.0	4.4 ± 0.3	245 ± 50	67.0 ± 7.7	1810 ± 222	1/6
p value AC	< 0.001	< 0.01	< 0.05	ns	< 0.01	ns	ns	ns
AE	< 0.001	< 0.001	< 0.01	ns	< 0.005	ns	ns	< 0.025
CE	< 0.01	< 0.01	ns	ns	ns	ns	ns	ns

tially they had marked loss of lean body mass and of total body nitrogen and potassium. When refed, muscle fatigue disappeared within 4 weeks and all functional abnormalities were restored by 8 weeks of refeeding, when the creatinine-height index was still very low at 67% and TBN had risen by only 13% (Figure 8-10). Interestingly, while their TBK and body fat had risen proportionately more during this period, they were still well below the level expected for their height. Despite an incomplete return to normal body composition, clinically these patients had restored their ability to exercise and function.

Muscle Biopsy Analysis in Malnutrition

In obese patients, fasting resulted in Type II fiber atrophy (78). In animals, 2–5 day fasting resulted in an increase in slow twitch oxidative fibers (Type I), but prolonged hypocaloric dieting resulted in the appearance of fibers depleted in both myosin and Na-K ATPase, a fiber type

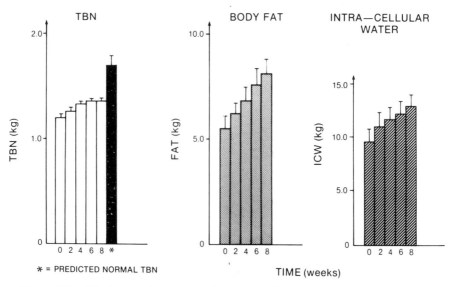

Figure 8-10. The bar graphs represent the mean ± SEM values for body composition at baseline assessment and following 2, 4, 6, and 8 weeks of oral refeeding of the six patients with anorexia nervosa noted in Figure 8-7. Baseline TBN was markedly depleted when compared with the predicted normal TBN. After 4 weeks of refeeding, TBN increased by only 10% (120g) and after 8 weeks by 13% (160g). Intracellular water (or TBK) rose by 19% after 4 weeks of refeeding, and by 32% after 8 weeks, while total body fat increased 48% (2.5 kg) after 8 weeks.

not normally seen (79). Despite these very different fiber type patterns, the muscle function abnormalities and fatigability were similar with nutritional deprivation.

The most striking finding during hypocaloric dieting and fasting in both humans and rats was an increase in the total water content, and an increase in both the intracellular concentration and total ionic content of muscle sodium and calcium. In contrast, total potassium, magnesium, chloride, and phosphate remained normal. Other notable changes were a fall in the ATP/ADP ratio, and a rise in the lactate/pyruvate ratio in hypocalorically fed rats and in humans.

Phosphofructokinase fell with short-term fasting while succinate dehydrogenase and acyl CoA dehydrogenase remained normal or rose, suggesting a change to more oxidative fibers with early starvation (80). However, prolonged hypocaloric feeding was followed by a reduction in phosphofructokinase, succinate dehyrogenase, and acyl CoA dehydrogenase.

These studies indicate that there is a lack of relationship between changes in lean body mass and body function. It is clear that the loss or restoration of lean body mass is not essential for the occurrence of the corresponding changes in muscle contraction-relaxation characteristics and endurance properties. Our findings are consistent with the somewhat similar data concerning morbidity and mortality mentioned earlier (4,6). Thus one may well question whether the demonstration of malnutrition should depend on changes in lean body mass, and conversely whether the restoration of lean body mass and improved nitrogen balance constitute the gold standards for good nutritional support. Our findings indicate that the failure to restore body nitrogen, observed in earlier studies, does not negate the fact that such support may have restored function.

What, then, are the possible causes of the improved function noted? An obvious explanation for slow relaxation is loss of fast twitch fibers (Type II). However, there are several reasons for doubting this hypothesis. First, it has been shown that the contraction characteristics of many different muscles of completely different fiber composition are the same (73). Second, these functional effects of short-term fasting (associated with maintenance of oxidative enzyme activity) are the same as after prolonged hypocaloric feeding (when all enzymes are reduced). Third, histochemical examination showed that the fiber type, after prolonged hypocaloric feeding, is unlike that of Type I fibers.

In contrast, the most consistent finding was an increase in intracellular sodium and calcium in all situations associated with increased fatigue, slower relaxation, and a rise in the percent maximum force attained at lower frequencies—another way of expressing slower relaxation. In striated muscle, the regulation of the cellular calcium content is critical for its kinetic properties (81). In ventricular myocardial muscle fibers, membrane currents are dependent on the sodium and calcium influx and efflux during depolarization and repolarization. Clearly the accumulation of intracellular muscle calcium will reduce the muscle relaxation rate and alter the contraction characteristics. This accumulation can also interfere with mitochondrial function and may explain the increased intracellular lactate/pyruvate ratio. Calcium accumulation may conceivably result from high intracellular sodium, preventing the sodium-calcium exchange necessary for efflux of calcium during repolarization. Limiting cell energy may also be a factor, and indeed the ATP/ADP ratio was lower in these muscles after nutritional deprivation.

In conclusion, although many interesting avenues need confirmation and exploration, there is sufficient evidence to suggest that in the adult human the adverse functional effects of malnutrition cannot be equated to, nor quantitated by, a simple loss of lean body mass. Furthermore, restoration of body function cannot be equated to "regrowth" of lean body mass assessed by a gain in body nitrogen or the attainment of a positive nitrogen balance. The changes in cellular electrolytes at a time of functional impairment need further study.

REFERENCES

1. L. D. MacLean, J. L. Meakins, K. Taguchi, J. P. Buignan, K. S. Philton, and J. Gordon, *Ann. Surg.*, **182**, 207 (1975).

2. J. L. Meakins, J. B. Pietsch, O. Bubenick, et al. *Ann. Surg.*, **186**, 241 (1977).

3. M. V. Kaminski, Jr, M. J. Fitzgerald, R. J. Murphy, et al. *J. P. E. N.*, **1**, 27 (1977).

4. J. L. Mullen, M. H. Gertner, G. P. Buzby, G. L. Goodhart, and E. F., Rosato, *Arch. Surg.*, **114**, 121 (1979).

5. J. L. Mullen, G. P. Buzby, D. C. Matthews, B. F. Smale, and E. F. Rosato, *Ann. Surg.*, **192**, 604 (1980).

6. J. M. Muller, C. Dienst, U. Brenner, and H. Pichlmaier, *Lancet*, **1**, 68 (1982).

7. M. A. Rothschild, M. Oratz, and S. S. Schreiber, Albumin Synthesis, in Javitt, Ed., *Liver and Biliary Tract Physiology*, Baltimore, University Park Press, 1980, pp. 249-274.

8. T. Peters, Jr. Serum Albumin, in Putman, Ed., *The Plasma Proteins. Structure, Function and Genetic Control*, Vol 1, 2nd ed, New York, Academic 1975, pp. 133-181.

9. D. A. Shafritz, *Gastroenterology*, **77,** 1335 (1979).

10. P. S. Shetty, R. T. Jung, K. E. Watrasiewicz, and W. P. T. James, *Lancet*, **2,** 230 (1979).

11. G. A. Young, J. P. Collins, and G. L. Hill, *Am. J. Clin. Nutr.*, **32,** 1192 (1979).

12. L. J. Berry and D. F. Rippe, *J. Infect. Dis.*, **128,** (suppl) S118 (1973).

13. K. N. Jeejeebhoy, *Lancet*, **1,** 343 (1962).

14. R. K. Chandra, *Br. Med. J.*, **3,** 608 (1974); *Br. Med. J.*, **2,** 583-85.

15. R. K. Chandra, *Clin. Exp. Immunol.*, **38,** 228 (1979).

16. K. M. Yamada and K. Olden, *Nature* (London), **275,** 179 (1978).

17. T. M. Saba and E. Jaffe, *Am. J. Med.*, **68,** 577 (1980).

18. D. F. Mosher, R. A. Proctor, and J. E. Grossman, Fibronectin: Role in Inflammation, in Weissman, Ed., *Advances in Inflammation Research*, Vol. 2, New York, Raven, 1981, pp. 187-207.

19. E. Ruoslahti, E. Engvall, and E. Hayman, *Collagen Res.*, **1,** 95 (1981).

20. T. M. Saba, B. C. Dillon, and M. E. Lanser, *J.P.E.N.*, **7,** 62 (1983).

21. M. E. Lanser, T. M. Saba, and W. A. Scovill, *Ann. Surg.*, **192,** 776 (1980).

22. W. A. Scovill, T. M. Saba, F. A. Blumenstock, et al., *Ann. Surg.*, **188,** 521 (1979).

23. H. McFarlane, *Adv. Clin. Chem.*, **16,** 153 (1973).

24. R. K. Chandra, *Br. Med. Bull.*, **37,** 89 (1981).

25. R. K. Chandra, *Bull. World Health Organ.*, **57,** 167 (1979).

26. S. Driezen, *Int. J. Vitamin Res.*, **49,** 220 (1978).

27. R. K. Chandra and D. H. Dayton *Nutr. Res.*, **2,** 721 (1982).

28. W. R. Biesel, R. Edelman, K. Nauss, and R. M. Suskind, *J.A.M.A.*, **245,** 53 (1981).

29. P. Twomey, D. Ziegler, J. Rombeau, *J.P.E.N.*, **6,** 50 (1982).

30. W. P. Reed, J. W. Olds, A. L. Kisch, *J. Infect. Dis.*, **125,** 398 (1972).

31. R. J. Mangi, J. C. Niederman, J. E. Kelleher, et al., *N. Engl. J. Med.*, **291,** 1149 (1974).

32. A. G., Mitchell, W. E. Nelson, and T. J. LeBlanc, *Am. J. Dis. Child.*, **49,** 695 (1935).

33. W. E. Bullock, *N. Engl. J. Med.*, **278,** 298 (1968).

34. J. L. Meakins, N. V. Christou, H. M. Shizgal, and L. D. MacLean, *Ann. Surg.*, **190,** 286 (1979).

35. W. E. C. Wilson, C. H. Kirkpatrick, and D. W. Talmage, *Ann. Int. Med.* **62,** 1 (1965).

36. V. K. Bansal, S. Popli, J. Pickering, et al., *Am. J. Clin. Nutr.*, **33,** 1608 (1980).

37. B. Straus, M. Berenyi, J. Ming-Huang, et al., *Dig. Dis.*, **16,** 509 (1971).

38. R. A. Fox, P. F., Scheuer, S. Sherlock, et al. *Gut*, **9,** 729 (1968).

39. B. H. Toh, I. C. Roberts-Thomson, J. D. Matthews et al., *Clin. Exp. Immunol*, **14,** 193 (1973).

40. N. Snyder, J. Bessoff, J. M. Dwyer, et al., *Dig. Dis.*, **23,** 353 (1978).

41. S. Meyers, D. B. Sachar, R. N. Raub, et al., *Gut*, **17,** 911 (1976).

42. D. B. Sachar, R. N. Taub, K. Ramachandar, et al., *Ann. N.Y. Acad. Sci.*, **278,** 565 (1976).

43. W. R. Thayer, B. Fixa, O. Komarkova, et al., *Dig. Dis.*, **23**, 337 (1978).

44. J. V. Jones, *Clin. Exp. Immunol.*, **2**, 477 (1967).

45. E. L., Chusid, R. Shah, and L. E. Siltzbach, *Am. Rev. Resp. Dis.*, **104**, 13 (1971).

46. R. A. Goldstein, B. W. Janicki, J. Mirro, et al., *Am. Rev. Resp. Dis.*, **117**, 55 (1978).

47. J. L. Meakins, A. P. McLean, R. Kelly, et al., *J. Trauma*, **18**, 240 (1978).

48. J. M. Hiebert, M. McGough, G. Rodeheaver, et al., *Surgery*, **86**, 242 (1979).

49. J. B. Pietsch, J. L. Meakins, and L. D. MacLean, *Surgery*, **82**, 349 (1977).

50. D. M. Ota, E. M. Copeland, J. N. Corriere, et al., *Surg. Gynecol. Obstet.*, **148**, 104 (1979).

51. M. Boeva, T. Donchev, R. Markova, et al., *Neoplasma*, **25**, 733 (1978).

52. A. C. Campbell, P. Hersey, I. C. M. MacLennan, et al. *Br. Med. J.*, **2**, 385 (1973).

53. A. B. Cosimi, F. H. Brunstetter, W. T. Kemmerer, et al., *Arch. Surg.*, **107**, 531 (1973).

54. W. M. Wara, T. L. Phillips, D. W. Wara, et al., *Am. J. Roentgenol.*, **123**, 482 (1975).

55. S. Bovornkitti, P. Knsadal, P. Sathirapat, et al., *Dis, Chest*, **38**, 51 (1960).

56. R. R. MacGregor, J. N. Sheagren, M. B. Lipsett, et al., *N. Engl. J. Med.*, **280**, 1427 (1969).

57. H. Mailbach and W. L. Epstein, *Int. Arch. Allergy*, **27**, 102 (1965).

58. J. Avella, H. J. Binder, J. E. Madsen, et al., *Lancet*, **1**, 624 (1978).

59. J. S. Goodwin. *Lancet*, **1**, 934 (1978).

60. R. O. Bicks and E. W. Rosenberg *Lancet*, **1**, 552 (1980).

61. R. L. Edwards, *Science*, **200**, 541 (1978).

62. H. Yazici, P. D. Saville, and E. D. Chaperon, *Clin, Res.*, **22**, 645a (1974).

63. D. L. Bruce and D. W. Wingard *Anesthesiology*, **34**, 271 (1971).

64. K. N. Jeejeebhoy, J. P. Baker, S. L. Wolman, D. E. Wesson, B. Langer, J. E. Harrison, and K. G. McNeill, *Am. J. Clin. Nutr.*, **35**, 1117 (1982).

65. G. R. Greenberg and K. N. Jeejeebhoy, *J.P.E.N.*, **3**, 427 (1979).

66. G. A. Young and G. L. Hill *Ann. Surg.*, **192**, 183 (1980).

67. J. P. Baker, A. S. Detsky, D. E. Wesson, S. L. Wolman, S. Stewart, J. Whitwell, B. Langer, and K. N. Jeejeebhoy, *New Engl. J. Med.*, **306**, 969 (1982).

68. R. A. Forse and H. M. Shizgal, *Surgery*, **86**, 17 (1980).

69. H. M. Shizgal, *Surg. Gynecol. Obstet.*, **152**, 22 (1981).

70. P. A. Merton, *J. Physiol.*, **123**, 553 (1954).

71. R. H. T. Edwards, A. Young, and G. P. Hosking, *Clin. Sci. Mol. Med.*, **52**, 283 (1977).

72. R. H. T. Edwards, *Clin. Sci. Mol. Med.*, **54**, 463 (1978).

73. J. Moxham, A. J. R. Morris, S. G. Spiro, et al., *Thorax*, **36**, 164 (1981).

74. C. M. Wiles, A. Young, D. A. Jones, et al., *Clin. Sci. Mol. Med.*, **56**, 47 (1979).

75. J. Lopes, D. McR. Russell, J. Whitwell, and K. N. Jeejeebhoy, *Am. J. Clin. Nutr.*, **36**, 602 (1982).

76. D. McR. Russell, L. A. Leiter, J. Whitwell, E. B. Marliss, and K. N. Jeejeebhoy, *Am. J. Clin. Nutr.*, **37**, 133 (1983).

77. D. McR. Russell, P. J. Prendergast, P. L. Darby, P. E. Garfinkel, J. Whitwell, and K. N. Jeejeebhoy. A comparison between muscle function and body composition in anorexia nervosa: the effect of refeeding. *Am. J. Clin. Nutr.* (in press).

78. D. McR. Russell, A. A. F. Sima, P. M. Walker, W. K. Tanner, J. Whitwell, E. B. Marliss, L. A. Leiter, and K. N. Jeejeebhoy. Metabolic and structural changes in muscle during hypocaloric dieting. *Am. J. Clin. Nutr.* (submitted).

79. H. L. Atwood, D. McR. Russell, T. Itakura, and K. N. Jeejeebhoy. Histochemical and electron microscopic changes in rat skeletal muscles during fasting and hypocaloric dieting. *Nerve and Muscle* (submitted).

80. D. McR. Russell, T. Itakura, H. L. Atwood, P. M. Walker, D. A. G. Mickle, and K. N. Jeejeebhoy. The effect of fasting and hypocaloric diets on the functional and metabolic characteristics of rat hind limb muscles, *Clin. Sci.* (in press).

81. H. Reuter, and H. Scholz, *J. Physiol.*, **264**, 17 (1977).

9

Nutrition and Aging

S. JAIME ROZOVSKI, Ph.D.

Institute of Human Nutrition, Columbia University College of Physicians and Surgeons, New York, New York

The 20th Century has witnessed an unprecedented steady increase in the segment of the population 65 years old and older (Figure 9-1) (1). This increase is due to a greater life expectancy over previous centuries, a change brought about by a host of factors, including better public health conditions and a dramatic improvement in both preventive and curative medicine. Interestingly, despite the substantial increase in life expectancy, during the last 200 years the maximum life span has not changed significantly. Thus, the observed increase in life expectancy means not that people are living longer but that more people are allowed to reach an old age. Ideally, survival curves should be such that all individuals would reach an age as close to maximal life span as possible and then die (Figure 9-2). This possibility, of course, assumes that life-threatening diseases are nonexistent.

In the United States approximately 11% of the total population, or about 24 million people, are over 65 years of age (2) (Figure 9-3). This age group is increasing at a rate faster than the rest of the population (Table 9-1). By the year 2030 a projected increase will bring the total to more than 50 million, or 20% of the population. The existence of such a large segment of elderly people will create new realities for many obvious social programs, including welfare, health costs, and nursing care, and will probably have far-reaching effects on politics, economics, and culture.

The anticipation of these impending changes, together with some of the present realities, have stimulated a great deal of research interest in aging as a sociocultural and biological phenomenon. Among the biologi-

137

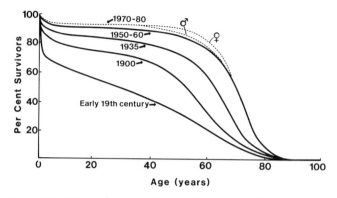

Figure 9-1. Human survivorship trends in the world population (1).

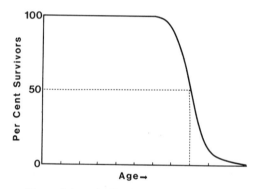

Figure 9-2. Idealized survivorship curve.

cal and biomedical aspects of aging, the role of nutrition has received special attention. Because of their unique and fundamental role in cell function, nutrients have been linked to the aging process. From a different perspective, because of chronic ailments, isolation, and low income, old people are susceptible to nutrient deficiency. Finally, aging is characterized by metabolic changes that may influence nutrient needs. Relatively little is known about these important aspects of the nutritional requirements of the elderly.

This chapter will analyze present knowledge of how nutrition is relevant to aging both as an intriguing biological process and as a human reality.

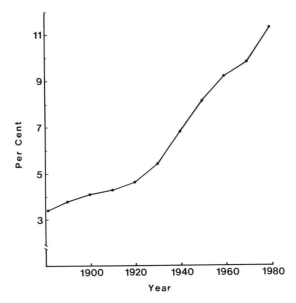

Figure 9-3. United States population age 65 and older as per cent of the total U.S. population.

Table 9.1   Percent Increase in Population (by decade) in the United States[a]

Population	1970–1980
Male	
65+	18.5
65–69	22.5
70–74	21.7
75+	11.7
Female	
65+	25.9
65–69	24.9
70–74	25.6
75+	26.9
Total Population	13.0

[a]Data from U.S. Census Bureau.

139

THEORIES OF AGING

Aging can be defined as a progressive and irreversible change which affects practically every system in the body and begins even before birth. The potential for maximum lifespan is genetically determined in an organism. Environmental factors, such as radiation, infections, and diet, influence the process of aging itself or the speed of this process. The precise time at which these factors act can also be important. The reason for aging is still unknown. Nevertheless several theories have been proposed.

The *waste product theory* postulates that metabolic "garbage" accumulates in the cells with aging. Lipofucsin, a yellow-brown intracellular pigment, has been found to accumulate in cells of different organs of elderly humans and old animals (3). The concentration of pigment is independent of sex and race and the rate of accumulation seems to increase linearly with age (4).

The *immunological theory* postulates that aging brings about an increasing immunogenetic diversification of the dividing cell population, leading to a loss of recognition patterns between the cells. This is manifested by autoimmune-like reactions (5,6).

The *mutation theory* postulates that deleterious effects may build up if spontaneous mutations accumulate in somatic cells (7). This theory has been partially supported by the observation that chromosomal aberrations increase with age (8).

The *free radical theory* postulates that the formation of free radicals damages tissues in a variety of ways, including lipid peroxidation (resulting in membrane alteration), breakdown of mucopolysaccharides, oxidative alteration of collagen, and other less specific modes (9,10). Certain inhibitors of free radical reactions have been found to increase the lifespan of mice when added to the diet. This will be discussed below.

The *wear and tear theory* postulates that stress will decrease life expectancy and presumably accelerate aging (11). However, there is no information available indicating whether stress per se causes aging, although it is quite obvious that the aged organism can withstand stress less than young ones.

The *collagen theory* postulates that the increase in collagen cross linking that occurs with age makes connective tissue become stiffer and more stable (12,13). This change may be responsible for the physical and mechanical changes observed in structures where collagen is present.

Recently a theory has developed based on the age-related changes in the comparison and morphology of mammalian membrane with age (14). Changes in membrane composition include alterations in the amount and the type of lipids in several organs of the rat and mouse and in human red blood cells. One aspect of the membrane hypothesis of aging involves a decrease in the resting potassium permeability of cellular membranes with aging due to increased rigidity (15). Although a discussion of the physiological effects of changes in the intracellular concentration of ions is beyond the scope of this chapter, it may have an important application in the study of nutrition and aging.

ALTERATION OF LIFESPAN BY NUTRITIONAL MANIPULATION

The role of nutrition in the aging process was called to the attention of the scientific community by McCay almost 50 years ago (16–18). The original investigations done by McCay and collaborators demonstrated that calorie restriction from early in life significantly prolonged life in rats. These studies have probably been a major factor contributing to the stimulation of research on the interrelationship between nutrition and aging. Other investigators have since extended these studies. Ross and Brass demonstrated that when rats were allowed to eat a balanced ad libitum diet an inverse relationship was found between food consumption and lifespan. Animals consuming the least food lived the longest (19).

The studies of Stuchlikova and co-workers have also shown that food restriction initiated in adult life will prolong life (20). In their studies food intake in rats was restricted at different ages (Table 9-2). If animals were restricted for the first 2 years of life they showed a significant increase in 50% survival. Survival improved when restriction was imposed only in the second year and the highest increase was found when restriction was imposed only in the first year of life. Other investigators have shown that altering proteins or carbohydrates in the diet can also alter lifespan (21,22). Even individual amino acids can create similar effects. Segall and Timiras showed that when rats are placed on a tryptophan-deficient but otherwise complete diet, an increase in both the maximum lifespan and in 50% survival occurs (23). The authors have proposed that lack of tryptophan delays the aging of the nervous system (24,25).

Table 9.2 Percent Increase in 50% Survival[a]

Restricted 1st year	33
Restricted 2nd year	
Ad libitum 1st year	43
Restricted 2nd year	
Restricted 1st year	61
Ad libitum 2nd year	

[a]Rats were restricted as indicated and compared with a group fed ad libitum throughout life. Adopted from Stuchlikova et al. (20).

What are the mechanisms by which dietary restriction increases longevity? Chronic restriction in animals decreases the incidence and severity of some diseases associated with aging including cancer (26–33). However, certain types of tumors, for example, epithelial carcinoma, have been shown to increase with dietary restriction (28). The normal aging of collagen also seems to be retarded during food restriction in rodents (34–36). Good and his collaborators showed that dietary restriction in mice delays the decline in thymus-dependent immunity and retards the appearance of autoimmune disease, preventing the immunological disorganization that normally occurs with aging (37).

These studies clearly indicate that diet has a major role in the process of aging. The human application of these findings still remains unclear. However, the elucidation of the mechanisms responsible for the increase in lifespan with dietary restriction may provide important clues for the study of aging.

PHYSIOLOGICAL CHANGES DURING AGING

The physiological alterations that occur during aging do not show a clear pattern of change. As shown in Figure 9-4, where changes in some selected functions are graphed as percent of values at age 30, certain functions, such as basal metabolic rate, show only a limited decrease with age. On the other hand others, such as maximal breathing capacity,

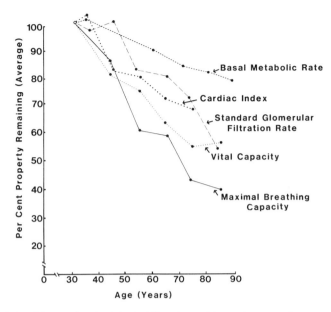

Figure 9-4. Changes in physiological functions with age (expressed as percent of mean values at age 30). Adapted from Shock (38).

show a 70–80% decrease from adult values (38). It is important to point out here that many physiological systems which show very little change with age are markedly affected when subjected to any stress.

Another important factor is that as age progresses the variability between individuals in a population increases. Undoubtedly this presents major problems when we try to set up guidelines to be applied to the elderly population.

Body composition changes progressively with aging. These changes include an increase of body fat, a decrease in body cell mass, and a decrease in bone mineral (39) (Figure 9-5). The decrease in lean body mass is progressive and is compensated by an increase in body fat (40,41).

The changes with aging in the gastrointestinal system may be the most important in terms of nutrition. It is general knowledge that the elderly cannot tolerate food as well as younger individuals. Although the data available are far from conclusive, some evidence both from observation in humans and from animal experimentation does indicate that gastro-

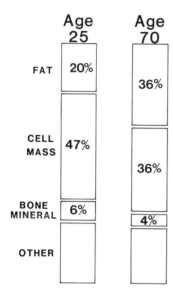

Figure 9-5. Differences in body composition with age in men. Adapted from Geigerman and Bierman (39).

intestinal function is impaired with age. The data have been recently reviewed by Holt (42).

A decrease in secretion of gastric acid with aging is well known. Furthermore, achlorhydria is estimated to occur in 24 to 65% of the aged population (43). The mechanisms responsible for the decrease in acid secretion are unknown. This condition may be due to a destruction of parietal cells, to diminished release of gastrin from these cells, or to reduced responsiveness of the parietal cell to gastrin (42). In general, there are no data related to changes in the hormonal responsiveness of the gastrointestinal tract with aging.

Aging reduces mucosal surface area (44) and villus height (45) in humans. The data are not conclusive and, in addition, studies in aged rats have shown that the number of intestinal crypts does not vary with age (46). Intestinal cell proliferation is decreased in aging animals (47) but no conclusive data on mucosal cell turnover in humans are available. Holt (42) has pointed out that the reference point used in calculating intestinal absorption is a major factor in studies in experimental animals. Changes in total absorption rates for a nutrient with aging calculated on the base of intestinal protein, intestinal length, or intestinal weight may give different results because of the different growth rates of these parameters with aging.

The absorption of certain nutrients is impaired with aging. The suggestion has been made that carbohydrate absorption in the elderly is altered, since in almost all cases older individuals show an abnormal oral glucose tolerance test (48,49). However, since the intravenous glucose tolerance test is also altered (50) factors other than glucose absorption may be responsible. Galactose (51), 3-methyl-glucose (52), and xylose (53) absorption have been shown to decrease with age, although more recently Montgomery and co-workers (54) showed that xylose absorption, once corrected for renal excretion, showed no correlation with age. Feibusch and Holt, using the technique of breath hydrogen analysis, showed that one-third of individuals beyond the age of 65 had some degree of carbohydrate malabsorption (55).

Protein absorption in the elderly has been studied only to a limited extent. Although some studies suggest that protein absorption may not differ in young and old subjects (56), no definite conclusions can be drawn at present (42).

Fat absorption is decreased in old age (57–59). However, many of these studies suggest that the decrease in absorption is due more to a decrease in pancreatic lipase production than in absorption per se (60).

The data on vitamin absorption in the elderly are equivocal. The problems inherent in performing proper studies involve poor methodology for determing vitamin intake and stores and for measuring direct vitamin absorption, human vitamin status, and so on. The data available suggest that aging produces a decrease in absorption of vitamins A, D, thiamine, and folic acid, although the results are not conclusive (42).

Mineral absorption is also impaired with age. Calcium absorption has been shown to be decreased in both humans (61–65) and rats (66–69). This decrease in calcium absorption with aging could be due to a decrease in responsiveness of the mucosal cell to 1,25 dihydroxycholecalciferol (42) or to a decreased formation of this hormone (70,71). The data available on changes in iron absorption with increasing age are more contradictory. While some studies report a decrease in absorption with age (72,73) other studies do not support these findings (74,75).

The results outlined above do point to the need of developing proper methodology to determine nutrient absorption in the elderly, which is of paramount importance in determining nutrient requirements in this sector of the population.

NUTRIENT REQUIREMENTS IN THE ELDERLY

Probably the area that deserves the most attention in the future with respect to nutrition for the elderly is related to the changes in nutrient requirements. What have mostly been used until now are extrapolations from observations performed in adults, which, in fact, may not be correct.

The elderly should be considered a different biological entity, as we do with the infant, the adolescent, or the adult. Many assume that an extrapolation from the adult, based on age changes, is sufficient when applied to the elderly. However, an individual who is 70 or 80 years old is different from an adult in many anatomical, physiological, and biochemical aspects. Although extrapolations in terms of requirements often attempt to take into consideration these changes, they often fail.

Studies of protein and amino acid requirements in the elderly have been quite controversial. This may reflect the almost impossible task of finding a group of "healthy" elderly without any complicating diseases. In addition race, sex, and geographical location may be important factors to consider. To complicate things further, the level of other dietary components (mainly energy) may play an important role in the outcome of clinical studies.

Body protein increases during early life to a peak at approximately 30 years of age in males and declines thereafter (76). In females the decline starts at about 40 years of age, but proceeds at a slower rate than in males (75). These studies have relied mainly in determination of ^{40}K as a reflection of lean body mass. Although the method is reliable, we do not have conclusive data on changes in intracellular potassium with aging.

Whole body protein synthesis and breakdown have been studied by Winterer and co-workers (78) at the Massachusetts Institute of Technology in young adults and elderly subjects ranging from 65 to 91 years of age using infusion of (^{15}N) glycine. Protein synthesis in elderly females was found to be significantly decreased. When synthesis is expressed per unit of body cell mass, determined by (^{40}K) counting or by unit of urinary creatinine excretion as an index of muscle mass, an increase in protein synthesis was observed for both males and females when compared with young adults (Figure 9-6).

A similar pattern of change was observed when protein breakdown was measured in these individuals (Figure 9-7). These data can be better

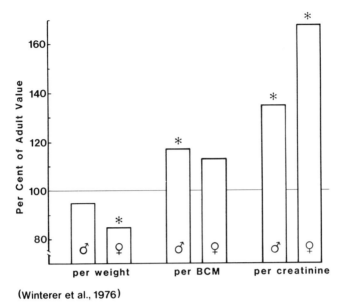

(Winterer et al., 1976)

Figure 9-6. Whole body protein synthesis in elderly males and females. Results are expressed as percent of adult values. *Significantly different from adult values. $p < 0.05$. Adapted from Winterer et al. (78).

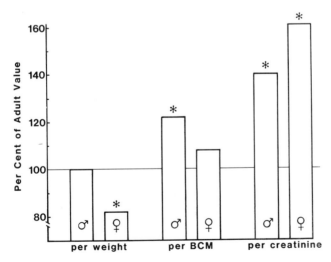

Figure 9-7. Whole body protein breakdown in elderly males and females. Values are expressed as percent of adult values. *Significantly different from adult values, $p < 0.05$. Adapted from Winterer et al. (78).

understood when one keeps in mind that the proportion of lean body mass decreases with age, which would explain the discrepancy depending on how the data are expressed.

Studies of albumin turnover are of interest since reduced albumin concentration is often found in aged people. Albumin levels have also been shown to be influenced by nutritional status (79–81). The reports on changes in albumin catabolism with aging have been controversial, showing either no change (82) or increased catabolism with age (83). Studies on albumin synthesis in older people have been very limited. In a recent study Gersovitz and co-workers (84), using (^{15}N) glycine, compared albumin synthesis in five young adults and six elderly males fed different amounts of dietary proteins. Serum albumin was lower in the elderly subjects regardless of the level of protein ingested. When dietary protein intake was reduced, serum albumin decreased in the old subjects while no change was observed in the young individuals. The fractional and absolute rate of albumin synthesis was not significantly different for young or old subjects at the high protein level (1.5 g/kg body weight). At the low protein level (0.4 g/kg body weight) the young subjects showed a significant decrease in albumin synthesis while the older individuals showed no change (Figure 9-8). The results are not conclusive because

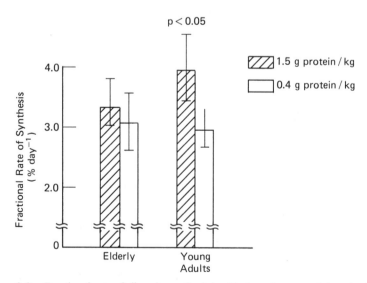

Figure 9-8. Fractional rate of albumin synthesis in elderly and young adult males fed two levels of dietary protein. Adapted from Gersovitz et al. (84).

of the small number of subjects employed and the use of a high protein diet containing twice the RDA for protein. However, they certainly indicate a difference in the liver's ability to synthesize and export albumin between young adults and older people. The authors propose that albumin synthesis in the elderly is controlled at a lower set point.

One of the most controversial aspects of the study of protein metabolism in the elderly is the determination of amino acid and total protein requirements. Studies of amino acid requirements have used several techniques, including balance, plasma amino acid response, excretion of urinary sulfate, and urinary amino acid excretion. Requirements for sulfur-containing amino acids have been shown to increase or decrease in the elderly when compared with the young adult (85). In these particular studies individual variations and the limited number of subjects utilized may account for the discrepancy. Using the plasma amino acid response, which is based on the principle that a reduced concentration of an amino acid in plasma reflects a deficient level of that amino acid in the diet, Young and his collaborators have concluded that requirements for essential amino acids may be higher in older individuals when compared with adults (85).

The problems in determining total protein requirements for the aged population are in part an extension of the dispute regarding protein allowances in the adult. The Recommended Dietary Allowances for protein are 56 g for adult men and 44 g for adult women, which corresponds to 0.8 g/kg body weight (86). These recommendations have been criticized as being too low. In addition, as is the case for other nutrients, they group all individuals above 51 years of age into one category.

The two methods currently utilized to measure protein requirements are the factorial method and the nitrogen balance method. Briefly, in the factorial method the individual is placed on a protein free but otherwise complete diet and the obligatory losses of nitrogen via urine and feces are determined after a stabilization period. Estimations are made for corrections for nitrogen losses through the skin and other routes. The sum of these nitrogen losses is considered the minimum requirement for maintenance. To correct for efficiency of utilization of protein 30% is added and an additional 30% is added to include variations found within the population.

Young and co-workers have suggested that the factorial method underestimates protein needs (85). One of the reasons for this could be the estimation of nitrogen losses through the skin and other minor routes. This additional loss, which is usually placed at 5 mg/kg body weight, can be much higher under certain conditions. The major assumption in this method is that the sum of the obligatory losses is equal to the minimum amount of nitrogen necessary to maintain nitrogen balance. This has proven not to be true, since it has been shown that higher amounts of good quality protein than that calculated by the factorial method are necessary to maintain nitrogen balance (85).

The nitrogen balance method measures the relationship between nitrogen ingested and nitrogen excreted. This method does not give an indication of internal distribution of tissue metabolism and, in addition, short-term studies can show a marked variability over a wide range of protein. In this method, as is the case in the factorial method, it is hard to quantitate all nitrogen losses, the previous protein intake may be a factor in results, and other dietary factors, mainly energy, can influence the results.

With the limitations of these methods in mind we can now look at some of the studies that have been done attempting to determine protein requirements in the elderly.

Investigations performed at the Massachusetts Institute of Technology have shown that the protein allowance calculated by the factorial method does not promote positive nitrogen balance in elderly volunteers (87). Investigators from the same group recently studied eight females and seven males ranging in age from 70 to 99 who were placed on a diet providing 0.8 g of egg protein/kg body weight/day for three consecutive periods of 10 days each (88). Nitrogen balance was determined for the last 5 days of each period. At the end of the first period, that is, after 10 days on the diet, all males were in negative nitrogen balance. After 30 days on the diet three of the seven subjects had not reached N equilibrium (Table 9-3). Similarly, at the end of the third period four of the eight females had not reached N equilibrium (Table 9-4). The authors further stress that since the diet used was based on a high quality egg protein this reinforces the view that a protein intake from mixed sources typical of the U.S. diet should actually be greater than 0.8 g/kg of body weight.

Although these data suggest that the current RDA for proteins is insufficient, other studies by Zanni and co-workers at the University of California (89) and by Cheng and co-workers at the University of Chile (90) showed opposite results. Cheng showed that most elderly subjects were kept in nitrogen balance when maintained on 0.8 g/kg body weight

Table 9.3 Nitrogen Balance (mg/kg/day); Protein Intake: 0.8g/kg/day—Males[a]

First	Second	Third
−16.1	− 2.1	1.7
− 1.5	0.1	13.5
− 0.9	18.6	− 2.7
− 1.3	11.6	3.6
−10.9	− 9.0	− 5.7
−12.1	− 3.6	−14.3
− 8.8	− 5.5	7.1

[a]From Gersovitz et al. (88).

Table 9.4 Nitrogen Balance (mg/kg/day); Protein Intake: 0.8g/kg/day—Females[a]

First	Second	Third
− 6.6	−11.0	3.9
11.5	−11.5	−13.0
0.5	−12.2	−14.0
0.8	− 8.5	2.5
− 4.2	− 5.4	2.2
0.8	1.9	6.9
− 3.6	− 4.6	−5.3
− 2.7	−10.8	−1.9

[a]From Gersovitz et al. (88).

for 11 days. Differences in the health status of the subjects in these studies, the level of protein in the diet previous to the study, and the level of energy intake during the studies may account for the differences between their results and those of other studies.

The studies described above stress the need for further research in the changes in protein requirements with aging. Although the technical difficulties are obvious there is a need for long-term, and carefully controlled balance studies. Other factors in the diet should also be carefully controlled, since changes in dietary energy can affect nitrogen balance. Stress, which has been shown to alter nitrogen balance in young individuals (91), can also markedly affect protein needs in the aged.

PROTEIN INTAKE AND CALCIUM METABOLISM

In recent years a relationship between dietary protein and certain aspects of calcium metabolism has been suggested. The studies of Linkswiler and collaborators have shown that increased dietary protein increases urinary calcium excretion in humans (92–96). Others have confirmed these observations (97,98).

Table 9-5 shows the results of a study where the same subjects were placed on diets providing 47 or 142 g/day of protein. After 10 days on the high protein diet there was an increase in urinary excretion of cal-

Table 9.5   Calcium Balance (mg/day) ($\bar{X} \pm$ SD)[a]

	Protein Intake (g/day)	
	47	142
Urinary Ca (mg/day)	150 ± 27	306 ± 47
Fecal Ca (mg/day)	381 ± 11	364 ± 38
Ca balance (mg/day)	−15 ± 31	−156 ± 65

[a]From Kim and Linkswiler (92).

cium which produced a negative calcium balance (92). Recent studies have shown that this increased urinary excretion also occurs in the elderly. Schuette and co-workers (99) showed that increasing protein intake from 42 to 112 g per day while maintaining calcium, magnesium, and phosphorus intake constant increased urinary calcium excretion and decreased calcium retention in males ranging from 44 to 86 years and females ranging from 65 to 79 years of age. In these studies the high level of protein in the diet was achieved by utilizing purified proteins.

In a study in which the high protein diet (2 g/kg body weight) was achieved by adding meat to the diet no change in calcium excretion was observed when calcium levels in the diet were low (200 mg/day) in males aged 40 to 67 years (Table 9-6) (100). At normal calcium levels (800 mg/day), there was on the average no increase in urinary calcium and the high excretion of calcium observed initially in two patients returned to normal after a few days. The authors proposed that the high phosphorus content of the meat diet is responsible for the lack of increase in calcium excretion.

Table 9.6   Calcium Balance and Urinary Excretion (mg/day) in Males[a]

	Balance	Urinary
Low Ca (200 mg)		
Control (0.9 g/kg)	−94 ± 22	93 ± 32
High protein (2 g/kg)	−82 ± 24	110 ± 27
Normal Ca (800 mg)		
Control	60 ± 14.9	113 ± 55
High protein	115 ± 36.5	107 ± 32

[a]From Spencer et al. (101).

The relation between dietary protein intake and calcium excretion should be further studied to establish whether the high protein intake may contribute to the incidence of osteoporosis in our elderly population.

OSTEOPOROSIS

A discussion of nutrients in relation to aging necessarily involves a discussion of osteoporosis. This condition is widespread in the elderly and is severe enough to result in vertebral, long bone, or hip fractures in 10% of the population over 50 years of age (101).

Cohn and co-workers have shown that the rate of loss of total body calcium increases markedly in elderly females when compared with young ones and have estimated that elderly females lose body calcium at a rate of 1% per year. The rate is higher in females than in males. From survey data it has been estimated that bone loss in individuals above 50 years of age ranges from 15 to 50% (101).

Osteoporosis has been developed in experimental animals placed on an otherwise complete but calcium deficient diet (103–105). The extrapolation of these studies to the human condition is difficult since studies of calcium intakes on osteoporotic patients have been contradictory (106–108). Nevertheless, data from several surveys do suggest a decreased calcium intake in the elderly (109,110). Calcium absorption has been reported to decrease with age in patients with osteoporosis (62,63,65,71) and in patients with osteoporosis compared to age-matched controls (111–114). In rats, the adaptive capability of the intestine to increase calcium absorption when intake is low has been shown to decrease with aging (115,116).

A probable explanation for this decrease in absorption appears to be a diminished conversion of 25-hydroxycholecalciferol (25-OH-D$_3$) to 1,25-dihydroxycholecalciferol (1,25-(OH)$_2$-D$_3$), the active form of vitamin D, in the aged kidney. This is derived from the findings of Gallagher and co-workers, (68,69) who have reported low levels of circulating 1,25-(OH)$_2$-D$_3$ in the serum of elderly subjects. A decrease in circulating 1,25-(OH)$_2$-D$_3$ and in the in vitro conversion of 25-(OH)-D$_3$ to 1,25-(OH)$_2$-D$_3$ by the kidney with aging has been shown in rats (117,118). A decrease in intestinal calcium binding protein has been shown to parallel the decline in calcium absorption (115,116,118). Other

Table 9.7   Changes After Administration of 0.5 μg
1,25-OH$_2$-D$_3$ ($\bar{X}$ ± SEM) in Elderly Females[a]

	Baseline	6–8 months
Ca absorption	7 ± 3%	27 ± 3%
Ca balance	−59 ± 22 mg/d	+2 ± 26 mg/d

[a]From Gallagher et al. (119).

studies in the elderly have shown also that the responsiveness of the intestine to vitamin D is diminished, which could be explained by a defect in the conversion of 25-(OH)D$_3$ to 1,25-(OH)$_2$-D$_3$ (63).

Recently, investigators from the University of Wisconsin treated a group of osteoporotic subjects either with 0.5 μg/day of 1,25-(OH)$_2$-D$_3$ or with placebo for from 6 to 8 months (119). After this period both calcium absorption and calcium balance showed substantial improvement in the treated patients but not in the placebo group (Table 9-7). Their results, although not conclusive, suggest an increase in bone volume with long-term therapy.

These data are exciting because they suggest possibiliites for the effective treatment of osteoporosis in the future. Further long-term studies in larger numbers of patients should be undertaken.

FIBER

Fiber is probably the most poorly defined component of the diet because it is composed of a wide variety of chemical entities. In general, fiber is divided into crude fiber and dietary fiber complex. Crude fiber is generally considered to be the structural matter of plants that remains after sequential extraction with dilute acid and dilute alkali. The dietary fiber complex, or more commonly dietary fiber, is often considered to be all matter resistant to the action of animal enzymes. This should include any portion of animal products that is resistant as a result of cross-linking or other chemical bonding.

The dietary components making up fiber are shown in Table 9-8. The method of analysis defines, for the most part, which of these will be included in reported values for fiber in any food table. A great deal of research has come from epidemiological studies, where inverse correla-

Table 9.8   Classification of Fiber by Structure[a]

Type	Chemical Component
Cellulose	Linear glucose polymer
Hemicellulose	Xylose, mannose, glucose, galactose
Pectin	Galacturonic acid
Gums	Galacturonic acid-rhamnose or mannose
Mucilages	Galactose-mannose
	Galacturonic acid-rhamnose
	Arabinose-xylose
Polysaccharides	Mannose, xylose, glucose, glucuronic acid
Lignin	Sinaply, confieryl, coumaryl alcohols

[a]Adapted from Kritchevsky (20).

tions between high intakes of fiber and the incidence of a series of diseases have been seen (120).

In the last 10 years a great deal of controversy has been generated over the role of fiber in the diet. Its lack has been implicated in a host of disorders, including chronic constipation, diverticular disease of the colon, carcinoma of the colon, cholelithiasis, hiatus hernia, hemorrhoids, appendicitis, diabetes, and coronary heart disease (120,121).

Reports show a decline in the intake of fiber from fruits and vegetables of about 20% in the last century in this country while that from cereals and grains has probably decreased approximately 50% (122). It is also known that the consumption of fiber-containing foods represents approximately 82% of the calories consumed in developing countries, compared to 32% in Western countries (123).

In the elderly the decrease in fiber intake is probably even greater since foods rich in fiber are usually hard to chew and difficult to digest. The fact that the elderly often cut the consumption of vegetables when having gastrointestinal problems may create additional problems, since an inverse relation has been noted between fiber intake and intestinal transit time and a direct relation between fiber intake and fecal weight (121). In recent years it has become obvious that the type of fiber may have different influences in these variables. Recently Spiller (125) and co-workers reported that cellulose did increase transit time whereas pectin did not. Therefore, caution must be exercized when generalizing about the effects of dietary fiber.

Diverticular disease of the colon probably accounts for disability in 5-10% of the over 60 population in this country although adequate surveys have not been performed. It is an age-related condition affecting 42% of the population over 80 and 19% of the population between 40 and 59. Its relationship to fiber intake is twofold. First, the incidence of the disease is lower in developing countries compared with Westernized societies (126). Some reports (127,128) have shown alleviation of symptoms of diverticular disease in patients treated with bran. The type of bran and the size of bran particles seem to be important in determining the effects. A weakness of many of these studies is that they were not conducted in a double-blind manner. In three double-blind studies the results were less conclusive. One study did find a beneficial effect of the addition of bran to the diet (129) while two other studies reported no difference (130,131). Observations derived mainly from epidemiological studies suggest that fiber may be protective against cancer of the colon, a disease whose frequency rises markedly beyond the age of forty. Nevertheless, the evidence is mainly indirect (132). Some data suggest that fiber may protect against coronary heart disease by lowering serum cholesterol and by affecting the absorption and metabolism of cholesterol. Again, these effects seem to be dependent on the type of fiber given (120). A similar situation is found in studies on the relationship between fiber and insulin requirements: while certain fibers, like bran, induce hypoglycemia, others can be hyperglycemic (133).

Overall, the evidence does point toward a need to increase the fiber intake of the entire population and especially of the elderly population as a preventive health measure, although in the majority of these disease processes a direct cause and effect relationship has not been demonstrated. The data also point toward a need to investigate altered responsiveness in young and old populations to both the beneficial effects of increased fiber intake and deleterious effects of reduced intake at the biochemical, physiological, and microbiological levels. As mentioned before, we have to be aware of the practical problems when increasing the fiber intake of the elderly.

NUTRITION AND THE THEORIES OF AGING

An exciting area that is developing in nutrition research concerns the possibility of using nutritional manipulation to delay processes that may be related to aging.

Table 9.9   Lipofuscin Pigment in Mice on a Protein-Restricted Diet[a]

Age (months)	Brain (% of control)	Heart (% of control)
3	71.3	97.5
5	60.9	89.5
7	82.1	96.2
12	48.2	74.7

[a]Control mice were kept on a 26% protein diet while restricted mice were kept on a 4% protein diet, both fed ad libitum. Table adapted from (134).

As was previously mentioned, it has been suggested that the accumulation of the pigment lipofucsin in cells with aging is involved in the aging process. When rodents were restricted in protein for prolonged periods of time a decrease in pigment concentration in liver, brain, and heart was observed when compared with control animals (Table 9-9) (134). Vitamin E deficiency has been shown to increase pigment accumulation, while addition of vitamin E decreases it (135-138). Although Csallany and co-workers have contested some of this study (139), problems in the methodology employed make it hard to draw definite conclusions (140).

Dietary restriction will also delay the immunological disorganization that occurs with aging, which has been proposed to be of relevance in the aging process (5,37,141).

The free radical theory of aging proposes that free radical formation would be expected to produce a series of deleterious effects that play an important role in the process of aging (142,143). Although an increased dietary intake of free radical promoters (like fat) has been shown to decrease life span in mice (144), the data are not clear with respect to the addition of natural antioxidants, such as vitamin C and vitamin E, to the diet (145). Although it is not clear now if the free radical theory will develop into a major cause of aging, further investigations into age-associated changes in vitamin E and ascorbic acid metabolism and their effects on free radical reactions seem warranted.

One of the theories of aging that has been developed in recent years is based on the age-related changes in the composition and morphology of mammalian membranes (14). These changes involve alterations in the morphology of plasma membrane in liver cells, in mitochondrial membrane, and in the endoplasmic reticulum. Changes in composition of the membrane in terms of total lipid or phospholipid have been demonstrated in several organs of the rat and mouse, and in human red blood cells. Phosphatidyl choline concentration has been shown to decrease and the cholesterol/phospholipid ratio to increase with aging in membranes from liver and muscle. A decrease in polyunsaturated fatty acids and an increase in monounsaturated fatty acids have also been reported to occur with aging (14,15).

One aspect of the membrane hypothesis of aging involves a decrease in the resting potassium permeability of cell membranes with aging due to an increased rigidity (15). In the past, several studies have dealt with the modification of plasma membranes by dietary manipulation. Studies in isolated cells showed that by increasing the concentration of polyunsaturated fatty acids in the medium, the proportion of polyunsaturated to saturated fatty acid in the cell membrane can actually be increased (148–149). In vivo studies altering the composition or quantity or both of fat in the diet have also shown alterations in the membrane lipid composition with a variety of different dietary lipids (150–155). The implications of these findings are obvious: If membrane changes are part of the aging process, what would happen when the composition of the membrane is changed by dietary manipulations? Can the aging process be altered by these experimental manipulations? We feel that more research in this area will lead to a better understanding of the mechanism by which aging occurs.

FOOD INTAKE IN THE ELDERLY

Several studies have shown that food intake decreases with aging. The reasons for this are multiple (Table 9-10). Denture problems, intestinal disorders, the presence of diseases like cancer, diabetes, and ulcers, and loss of memory are some of the factors responsible. Loneliness also decreases the individual's interest in preparing nutritious meals (156).

Although reports of studies of dietary intake in the elderly have increased notably in the last decade, they have been undertaken with less frequency than for other age groups. One of the most important problems in assessing the dietary intake in the elderly population is the methodology employed in these surveys.

Table 9.10   Causes of Inadequate Nutrition in the Aged

Organic
　Poor denture
　　Gastrointestinal disorders and malabsorption
　　Presence of disease
　　Mental deterioration

Psychosocial
　Apathy
　Loneliness
　Depression

Physical disability
Inadequate nutrition knowledge
Poverty

The methods usually employed to collect data on nutrient intake of a population include dietary histories, 24-hour recalls, and food records (109). This latter method, which involves recording or weighing intake of foods, requires a high degree of cooperation from the subjects. It may be too limited in terms of the days when the record can be taken, and is cost ineffective.

Dietary histories and 24-hour recalls rely to a high degree on the memory of the individual interviewed. Therefore, the accuracy of these methods when applied to the elderly has to be looked upon critically, considering the decrease in recall memory with aging (157). Several studies suggest that the 24-hour recall method is likely to overreport low intakes and underreport high intakes (158). In addition a substantial amount of nutrients can be "probed" by questioning (159). This seems to be particularly true in the case of calories in the elderly individuals (109). Nevertheless, the 24-hour recall is still a relatively simple way of obtaining information.

Dietary histories are usually based on food frequencies with questions asked in reference to general food patterns for a period of time up to one year. This method is time-consuming but it accounts for seasonal variation and can readily identify an individual that is consuming a fad diet or diets that exclude one or more important foods. Dietary histories have been reported to overestimate protein intakes (160).

The methods described above have obvious advantages and disadvantages when applied to the elderly. As mentioned above, this population group is particularly prone to present deficiencies in memory recall and have diseases that could cause modification of the diet, for example, ulcers and diabetes. In addition, the apathy toward the environment and other individuals often seen in the aged can markedly affect the outcome of dietary interviews. These are issues that should be taken into account in any study of nutrient intake. The development of proper interviewing methods to circumvent them is very desirable.

A source of confusion often encountered when evaluating surveys of dietary intake in the elderly is the different standards used. The most commonly used standard in dietary surveys is the Recommended Dietary Allowances (RDA) of the National Research Council-National Academy of Sciences. However, continuous revision of this standard has changed the level of adequate intake of particular nutrients. The latest RDA (84) shows a decrease in energy requirement for people above 76 years of age when compared with the previous RDA (152), which grouped all people over 51 years of age. In general, these continuous revisions have lowered protein, energy, and vitamin C recommendations. Many of the surveys have used different proportions of the RDA as their standard of adequate intake, which can alter the interpretation of results.

Several large dietary surveys have been performed in the aged U.S. population (109). These include the Ten-State Nutrition Survey (162), the Household Food Consumption Survey (163), and the Health and Nutrition Examination Survey (HANES) (155). In addition, dietary surveys have been performed in smaller groups involving people in nursing homes, in senior housing, and in free-living conditions.

Energy intake has often been found to be inadequate in the elderly. The national surveys found deficiencies in the caloric intake of the elderly population. The deficiencies were even more accentuated in individuals below the poverty level (109). Some particular groups, for example, Hispanics in low income states, were markedly deficient in their caloric intake. It is important to remember that these figures represent average intakes and they give no indication of individuals consuming extremely low or high amounts of calories. It is also curious that several surveys have reported decreased caloric intakes in groups that show a substantial prevalence of obesity. This discrepancy could be due to underreporting of calories. In more controlled studies the proportion of elderly consuming below standard for calories was much less than that in larger national surveys (165).

Protein intake of the elderly has been found to be adequate in most surveys, with the exception of the Ten State Nutrition Survey. This survey, which used as a standard intake 1 g of protein per kg body weight per day (higher than the RDA of 0.8 g/kg/day) found intakes below their standard in males and females in the low income states. The data on protein intake must be viewed with caution since the controversy about requirements still persists. In addition, the information obtained does not give an idea of the quality of protein consumed. Protein deficiency has been reported in some limited studies in low income groups (109).

Vitamin A intake was found to be low in 20% of women and 15% of men over 65 using two-thirds of the RDA as a standard. The low intake was more prevalent in Spanish-American individuals.

Several reports have shown adequate intake of ascorbic acid in subjects above 65 but others have given conflicting results. At least one-third of subjects in the Ten State Nutrition Survey had intakes below the standard of 30 mg per 1000 calories/day.

Thiamin consumption has been shown to be adequate in many surveys although in the Ten State Nutrition Survey about one-third of individuals were shown to be consuming less than their standard of 0.4 mg/1000 calories. The reason for these conflicting results is not clear.

The data on riboflavin and folic acid intake are controversial since some surveys have reported them be low, whereas other studies do not support these observations (109).

Calcium intake has been found to be low in many studies, the problem being more prevalent in women than in men, even when two-thirds of the RDA, that is, 533 mg/day, was used as a standard. This mineral is one of the nutrients most often deficient in the elderly.

Iron intake has been found to be low in several surveys of the elderly. The Health and Nutrition Examination Survey reported 26% of the over 65 population consuming less than two-thirds of the RDA. Low intakes are more prevalent in women than in men.

The data on nutrient intake in the elderly must be looked upon cautiously. What we usually see is the mean intake of the group and very often no idea is given of the variation in intake between individuals in any given group. For instance, in one study 73 elderly subjects were reported consuming on the average 0.9 g of protein per kilogram of body weight, which is more than adequate according to the current RDA standard (166). However, intake in these individuals ranged from 0.4 to 1.8 g/kg of body weight.

STUDIES IN OUR LABORATORY

In recent years we have become interested in the effect of long-term malnutrition on the organism. We have previously described cyclical changes in the synthesis of RNA and the synthesis and concentration of polyamines in the liver of young adult rats placed on a protein-deficient (6%) diet (167,168). These changes involve an initial increase in the activity of ornithine decarboxylase and s-adenosylmethionine decarboxylase, and in the concentration of the polyamines putrescine and spermidine, as well as in the activity of nucleolar DNA dependent RNA polymerase. When malnutrition was prolonged all these variables returned to normal (Figure 9-9). We have interpreted these results as a process of adaptation to malnutrition in which the organism initially attempts to preserve certain indispensable functions at the expense of dispensable functions (for instance, growth). Once this is accomplished and the requirements are reduced by the cessation of growth, RNA and polyamine synthesis return to normal (169). More recently we have performed similar studies in protein-deficient 24-month-old rats. The

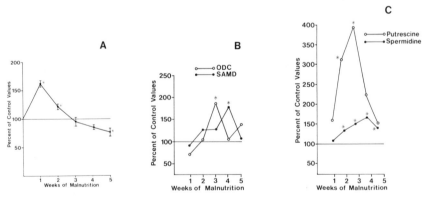

Figure 9-9. Neucleolar DNA-dependent RNA polymerase activity (dpm/mg protein) A. L-ornithine decarboxylase and s-adenosylmethionine activity (pmole CO_2/30 min/mg protein) and B. polyamine concentration (mmole/mg DNA) in young adult rats fed a 6% casein diet. Values are expressed as percent of values obtained from control rats fed a 25% casein diet. Each point represents the mean of at least six animals. *Significantly different from controls, $p < 0.05$.

model of protein malnutrition used in these studies is one that we have established previously, that is, feeding a 3.0% protein diet ad libitum. This diet produces cellular changes in the old animal that are qualitatively and quantitatively similar to the ones observed in young adult rats fed a 6% protein diet (a diet containing 6% protein does not produce any significant cellular changes in aged rats (S. J. Rozovski and M. E. Temkin, unpublished results). When the old animals were placed on the 3.0% protein diet the activity of ornithine decarboxylase initially increased (as we had observed in young animals) but it remains elevated without returning to normal (Figure 9-10) (S. J. Rozovski and S. M. Abrams, unpublished results). These results suggest that the aged animal cannot adapt as the young animal does. We are currently investigating whether the old rats take longer to adapt or, in fact, never do adapt.

We have expanded these studies on the effect of protein deficiency on the aged organism to certain aspects of energy metabolism and thermoregulation (170,171). We have recently showed that when an old

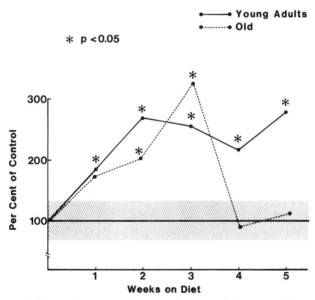

Figure 9-10. Activity of ornithine decarboxylase (pmole/mg protein/60 minutes) in young adult (dashed line) and 24-month-old (continuous line) rats placed on a 6% or a 3% protein diet, respectively. Both groups are compared to aged matched controls fed a 22% protein diet. *Significantly different from age matched controls, $p < 0.05$.

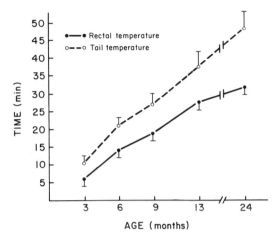

Figure 9-11. Changes in recovery time in rectal and tail temperature after a mild cold challenge with age in rats.

animal is exposed to mild cold it has more difficulty maintaining body temperature than a younger one. In addition, it takes longer for the old animal to return body temperature to normal after a mild cold challenge than a young one (Figure 9-11). Protein-deficient young rats show similar results when exposed to a mild cold challenge, when compared with well-nourished animals. It would be expected then that an aged protein-deficient rat will show an even more impaired response. We are currently investigating this aspect.

Some information contained in this review was extracted from the report "Nutrition in the Elderly" by S. J. Rozovski, M. W. Hamm, and M. Winick, prepared for the ITT Continental Baking Company's Program of Nutrition for Older Americans. Support for some of the work presented here was provided by a grant from ITT Continental Baking Company's Program of Nutrition for Older Americans. I would also like to thank Ms. Carol Rinko and Ms. Jan Kasofsky for their help in the preparation of this manuscript, and Mrs. Harriet Jacoby for typing and putting the manuscript together.

REFERENCES

1. B. L. Strehler, *Fed. Proc.*, **34,** 5 (1975).
2. U.S. Census Bureau.
3. B. L. Strehler, D. D. Mark, A. S. Mildran, and M. V. Gee, *J. Gerontol.*, **14,** 430 (1959).

77. G. B. Forbes and J. C. Reina, *Metabolism,* **19,** 653 (1970).

78. J. C. Winterer, W. P. Steffee, W. Davy, et al., *Exp. Gerontol.,* **11,** 17 (1976).

79. H. N. Munro, C. Hubert, and B. S. Baliga, "Regulation of Protein Synthesis in Relation to Amino Acid Supply. A Review," in M. A. Rothschild, M. Oratz, and S. Schreiber, Eds., *Alcohol and Abnormal Protein Synthesis,* New York, Pergamon, 1975, pp. 33-66.

80. M. A. Rothschild, M. Oratz, and S. S. Schreiber, *Ann. Rev. Med.,* **26,** 91 (1975).

81. G. Schreiber and J. Urban, *Rev. Physiol. Biochem. Pharmacol.,* **82,** 27 (1978).

82. A. S. Yan and J. J. Franks, *J. Lab. Clin. Med.,* **72,** 449 (1968).

83. D. P. Misra, J. M. Loudon, and G. E. Staddon, *J. Gerontol.,* **30,** 304 (1975).

84. M. Gersovitz, H. N. Munro, J. Udall, and V. R. Young, *Metabolism,* **29,** 1075 (1980).

85. V. R. Young, W. D. Perera, J. C. Winterer, and N. S. Scrimshaw, in M. Winick, Ed., *Nutrition and Aging,* New York, Wiley, 1976, p. 77.

86. Recommended Dietary Allowances, Food and Nutrition Board, National Academy of Sciences, Washington, D.C., 1980.

87. R. Uauy, N. S. Scrimshaw, and V. R. Young, *Am. J. Clin. Nutr.,* **31,** 779 (1978).

88. M. Gersovitz, K. Motil, H. N. Munro, N. S. Scrimshaw, and V. R. Young, *Am. J. Clin. Nutr.,* **35,** 6 (1982).

89. E. Zanni, D. H. Calloway, and A. Y. Zezulka, *J. Nutr.,* **109,** 513 (1979).

90. A. H. R. Cheng, A. Gomez, J. G. Bergan, T-C. Lee, F. Monckeberg, and C. O. Chichester, *Am. J. Clin. Nutr.,* **31,** 12 (1978).

91. N. S. Scrimshaw, J. P. Habicht, M. L. Piche, B. Sholskow, and G. Arroyave, *Am. J. Clin. Nutr.,* **18,** 321 (1966).

92. Y. Kim and H. M. Linkswiler, *J. Nutr.,* **109,** 1399 (1979).

93. N. E. Johnson, E. N. Alcantara, and H. M. Linkswiler, *J. Nutr.,* **100,** 1425 (1970).

94. R. M. Walker and H. M. Linkswiler, *J. Nutr.,* **102,** 1297 (1972).

95. C. R. Anand and H. M. Linkswiler, *J. Nutr.,* **104,** 695 (1974).

96. H. M. Linkswiler, C. L. Joyce, and C. R. Anand, *Trans. N.Y. Acad. Sci.,* Series II, **36,** 333 (1974).

97. S. Margen, J. Y. Chu, N. A. Kaufmann, and D. H. Calloway, *Am. J. Clin. Nutr.,* **27,** 524 (1974).

98. L. H. Allen, E. A. Oddoye, and S. Margen, *Am. J. Clin. Nutr.,* **32,** 741 (1979).

99. S. A. Schuette, M. B. Zemel, and N. M. Linkswiler, *J. Nutr.,* **110,** 305 (1980).

100. H. Spencer, L. Kramer, D. Osis, and C. Norris, *Am. J. Clin. Nutr.,* **31,** 2167 (1978).

101. A. A. Albanese, *Nutrition for the Elderly,* New York, Alan R. Liss, 1980, p. 187.

102. S. H. Cohn, A. Vaswani, I. Zanzi, J. F. Aloia, M. S. Roginsky, and K. J. Ellis, *Metabolism,* **25,** 85 (1976).

103. M. Harrison and R. Fraser, *J. Endocrinology,* **21,** 197 (1960).

104. R. F. Light and C. N. Frey, *Proc. Soc. Exp. Biol. Med.,* **48,** 256 (1941).

105. N. H. R. El-Maraghi, B. S. Platt, and R. J. C. Stewart, *Br. J. Nutr.,* **19,** 491 (1965).

106. R. W. Smith, W. R. Eyber, and R. C. Mellinger, *Ann. Int. Med.,* **52,** 773 (1960).

107. O. B. Hayes, L. J. Bowser, and M. F. Trulson, *J. Gerontol.,* **11,** 154 (1956).

108. R. W. Smith and B. Frame, *New Engl. J. Med.,* **273,** 73 (1965).

109. P. O'Hanlon and M. B. Kohrs, *Am. J. Clin. Nutr.*, **31**, 1257 (1978).

110. A. A. Albanese, in A. A. Albanese and D. Kritchevsky, Eds., *Current Topics of Nutrition and Diseases*, Vol. I, New York, Alan R. Liss, 1977.

111. A. Caniggia, C. Gennari, V. Bianchi, and R. Guideri, *Acta Med. Scand.*, **173**, 613 (1963).

112. V. R. Kinney, W. N. Tauxe, and W. H. Dearing, *J. Lab. Clin. Med.*, **66**, 187 (1966).

113. J. Szymendera, R. P. Heaney, and P. D. Saville, *J. Lab. Clin. Med.*, **79**, 570 (1972).

114. J. C. Gallagher, J. Aaron, A. Horsman, et al., *Clin. Endocrinol. Metab.*, **2**, 293 (1973).

115. H. J. Armbrecht, T. V. Zenzer, and M. E. H. Bruns, *Am. J. Physiol.*, **236**, E 769 (1979).

116. H. J. Armbrecht, T. V. Zenzer, C. J. Gross, and B. B. Davis, *Am. J. Physiol.*, **239**, E 322 (1980).

117. R. W. Horst, H. F. DeLuca, and N. Jorgenson, *Metab. Bone Dis. Rel. Res.*, **1**, 29 (1978).

118. H. J. Armbrecht, T. V. Zenzer, and B. B. Davis, *J. Clin. Invest.*, **66**, 1118 (1980).

119. J. C. Gallagher, C. M. Jerpbak, W. S. S. Jee, K. A. Johnson, H. F. DeLuca, and B. L. Riggs, *Proc. Natl. Acad. Sci.*, **79**, 3325 (1982).

120. D. Kritchevsky, *Bull. N.Y. Acad. Med.*, **58**, 230 (1982).

121. T. Almy, in M. Winick, Ed., *Nutrition and Aging*, New York, Wiley, 1976, p. 155.

122. J. Scala, *Food Technology*, **28**, 34 (1974).

123. H. Trowell, *Nutr. Rev.*, **35**, 6 (1977).

124. D. P. Burkitt, A. R. P. Walker, and N. S. Painter, *Lancet*, **2**, 1408 (1972).

125. G. A. Spiller, M. C. Chernoff, R. A. Hill, et al., *Am. J. Clin. Nutr.*, **33**, 754 (1980).

126. J. A. Kyle, D. Adesola, C. F. Tinekler, and deBeaux, *Scand. J. Gastroent.*, **2**, 77 (1967).

127. J. M. Findlay, A. N. Smith, N. D. Mitchell, *et al.*, *Lancet*, **1**, 146 (1974).

128. N. S. Painter and D. P. Burkitt, *Clin. Gastroenterol.*, **4**, 3 (1975).

129. A. J. M. Brodibb and D. M. Humphreys, *Brit. Med. J.*, **1**, 424 (1976).

130. C. Lyford, J. Fisher, B. Buess, et al., *Clin. Res.*, **23**, 253A (1975).

131. J. E. Soltoft, E. Gudman-Hoyer, E. Kristensen, and H. R. Sulff, *Lancet*, **1**, 270 (1976).

132. D. Kritchevsky and J. A. Story, in M. Winick, Ed., *Nutrition and Cancer*, New York, Wiley 1977, p. 41.

133. D. B. Jeffreys, *Proc. Nutr. Soc.*, **33**, 11A (1974).

134. H. Enesco and P. Kruk, *Exp. Gerontol.*, **16**, 357 (1981).

135. T. Moore and Y. L. Wang, *Br. J. Nutr.*, **1**, 53 (1947).

136. C. Raychaudhuri C. and Z. E. Desai, *Science*, **173**, 1028 (1971).

137. K. Reddy, B. Fletcher, A. Tappel, and A. L. Tappel, *J. Nutr.*, **103**, 908 (1973).

138. I. D. Desai, B. L. Fletcher, and A. L. Tappel, *Lipids*, **10**, 307 (1973).

139. A. S. Csallany, K. L. Ayaz, and L-C. Su *J. Nutr.*, **107**, 1792 (1977).

140. J. H. Shimasaki, N. Ueta, and O. S. Privett, *Lipids*, **17**, 878 (1982).

141. R. H. Weindruch, J. A. Kristie, and R. L. Walford, *Fed. Proc.*, **38**, 2077 (1979).

142. G. A. Sacher, in C. E. French and L. Hayflick, Eds., *Handbook of the Biology of Aging*, New York, Van Nostrand Reinhold, 1977, p. 582.

143. D. J. Harman, *Gerontol.*, **26**, 451 (1971).

144. D. J. Harman, *Am. Coll. Nutr.*, **1**, 27 (1982).

145. L. H. Chen, M. S. Lee, W. F. Hsing, and S. J. Chen, *Intl. J. Vit. Nutr. Res.*, **50**, 156 (1980).

146. A. L. Tappel, *Am. J. Clin. Nutr.*, **23**, 1137 (1970).

147. V. H. Engelhard, J. D. Esko, D. R. Storm, and M. Glasser, *Proc. Natl. Acad. Sci.*, **73**, 4482 (1976).

148. B. H. Ginsberg, T. J. Brown, I. Simon, and A. A. Spector, *Diabetes* **30**, 773 (1981).

149. R. McGee, *Biochem. Biophys. Acta.*, **663**, 314 (1981).

150. L. Rathbone, *Biochem. J.*, **97**, 620 (1965).

151. M. E. King, B. W. Stevens, and A. A. Spector, *Biochem.*, **16**, 5280 (1971).

152. B. P. Yu, F. A. Kummerow, and T. Nishika, *J. Nutr.*, **89**, 435 (1966).

153. G. A. Rao, K. Siler, and E. C. Rarkin, *Lipids*, **14**, 30 (1978).

154. D. E. Brenneman and C. O. Rutledge, *Brain Res.*, **179**, 295 (1979).

155. W. M. Tsang, J. Belim, and A. D. Smith, *Br. J. Nutr.*, **43**, 367 (1980).

156. J. Pelcovitz, *J. Am. Diet. Assoc.*, **60**, 297 (1972).

157. V. A. Kral, C. Cahn, and Mueller, *J. Amer. Geriat. Soc.*, **12**, 101 (1964); D. B. Bromley, *J. Gerontol.*, **13**, 398 (1958).

158. M. Gersovits, J. P. Madden, and H. Smicklas-Wright, *J. Am. Diet. Assoc.*, **73**, 49 (1978).

159. V. A. Campbell and M. C. Dodds, *J. Am. Diet. Assoc.*, **51**, 29 (1967).

160. J. Marr, *World Rev. Nutr. Diet.*, **13**, 105 (1971).

161. Recommended Dietary Allowances, National Academy of Sciences, Washington, D.C. 1974.

162. Ten State Nutrition Survey 1968-1970, V, Dietary, DHEW Publ. No. (HSM) 72-8133, U.S. Dept. of Health Education and Welfare, 1972.

163. U.S.D.A. Household Food Consumption Survey 1965-66, Food and Nutrient Intake of Individuals in the United States, Dept. No. 11, Washington, D.C., U.S. Printing Office, 1972.

164. First Health and Nutrition Examination Survey 1971-72, Preliminary Findings, Dietary Intake and Biochemical Findings, DHEW Publ. No. (HRA) 74-1219, Washington, D.C.

165. E. S. Yearick, M. S. L. Wang, and S. J. Pisias, *J. Gerontology*, **35**, 663 (1980).

166. V. E. Jordan, *Am. J. Clin. Nutr.*, **29**, 522 (1976).

167. S. J. Rozovski, P. Rosso, and M. Winick, *J. Nutr.*, **108**, 1680 (1978).

168. S. J. Rozovski, C. G. Lewis, and M. Cheng, *J. Nutr.*, **112**, 920 (1982).

169. S. J. Rozovski, and M. Winick, in M. Winick, Ed., *Nutrition Pre- and Postnatal Development*, New York, Plenum, 1979, p. 61.

170. T. Balmagiya and S. J. Rozovski, *Exp. Gerontol.*, **18**, 199 (1983).

171. T. Balmagiya and S. J. Rozovski, *J. Nutr.*, **113**, 228 (1983).

10

Nutrition, Diet, and Cancer—an Evaluation

ERNST L. WYNDER, M.D.

American Health Foundation, New York, N.Y.

The report by the National Academy of Sciences Committee on Nutrition, Diet, and Cancer has considered the present evidence in this field, reached a number of conclusions, and made specific recommendations (1). The report includes a careful overview of the literature detailing the state of knowledge of dietary components. The Committee had opportunity to consider a diverse set of data and opinions before making its decisions and preparing the interim dietary guidelines. As always in a scientific debate, there are opposing views as summarized by the Council for Agricultural Science and Technology (2). To the extent that some of the Committee's conclusions affect specific food categories, it can be readily understood that the producers of such foods find criticism and concern with the Academy report. Yet, and this is the value of an objective scientific debate, the facts based upon detailed scientific scrutiny from carefully structured research in man through epidemiology and metabolic epidemiology, and through laboratory research in model systems, have to prevail.

It is not within the purview of this chapter to review all of the evidence described in the Academy report. We shall cover the highlights and refer to the report for further details (1).

Proof for causality of noncommunicable chronic diseases was well described in the first Surgeon General's report *Smoking and Health* (3). This report and subsequent reports have delineated the diverse lines of evidence derived from epidemiology and other human studies, through experiments in animal models, as well as through specific experiments at the molecular level that smoking is associated with specific diseases (3).

Using a parallel approach, we shall develop the evidence supporting the working hypothesis that nutritional factors in general, and fats and fiber in particular, affect the incidence of several types of major human cancers. We will deal principally with the best-documented evidence for the relation of nutrition to breast and colon cancer for which fat (and fiber for colon cancer) is a key element. At the American Health Foundation, studies are carried forward with human subjects, and in animal models and in vitro systems, investigating the mechanisms of carcinogenesis in specific target organs such as the breast and colon. The study of cancer causation necessarily involves a search in the human setting for the relevant genotoxic carcinogens as well as for the nutritional modifiers affecting such genotoxic carcinogens. Another approach is to delineate the existence of promoting substances and, in particular, to establish the mechanisms whereby fat and fiber determine the risk for certain cancers.

Data derived from epidemiologic associations observed in humans and from animal experiments are so strongly suggestive of a causal relationship between cancer of the breast and colon and dietary fat intake that, although not ironclad, this association is strong enough to provide the basis for action and intervention. Considering the consequences of not acting, and thus maintaining the status quo in disease incidence, it is better to make sensible dietary changes rather than accept our diet as the best of all possible diets. This is especially true since such actions will not impose additional health risk to the public.

GENOTOXIC CARCINOGENS

At this time it is difficult to pinpoint a direct influence of a specific genotoxin in the customary food supply in Western countries. Although there are many naturally occurring carcinogens, their concentration in human food is usually low. The only carcinogen established to contribute to human cancer is aflatoxin, which has been shown to relate to the incidence of primary liver cancer in parts of Africa and Asia, perhaps in association with hepatitis B antigen (4–6). However, this does not seem to be the case in developed societies, such as the United States, where levels of aflatoxin in crops are now carefully monitored (7).

Contaminants of food, such as some of the other mycotoxins and N-nitroso compounds, have been found to be carcinogenic in animals, but there is a lack of evidence whether they would significantly contribute to human cancer risk, except perhaps for head and neck and gastric cancer. There are also insufficient data for studies in humans for other naturally occurring food components carcinogenic in laboratory animals, such as hydrazines, safrole, cycasin, or pyrrolizidine alkaloids. However, such compounds occur in the average U.S. diet in very small amounts. There is no evidence as to how much the polycyclic aromatic hydrocarbons present in the concentrations found in the dietary environment, including charcoal-cooked meats or smoked foods, contribute to total cancer risk.

It does not make sense to think that diethylstilbestrol (DES) in the concentration of the residues found in meat has a measurable impact on human carcinogenesis. Diethylstilbestrol is found in beef liver at 2 parts per billion, or 40 ng per serving. This quantity is distinctly different from the huge doses (50 million ng) given pregnant women in the 1950s that later resulted in the development of vaginal adenocarcinoma in daughters. No physiological significance or health effects are thus likely to result from the insignificant amount of DES found in meat (8, 9).

N-nitroso compounds (nitrosamines) are an important class of environmental carcinogens that might contribute to the total carcinogenic load, since many of them have caused tumors in experimental animals. These suspect compounds can be formed endogenously from ubiquitous prescursors. Exposure to nitrates, nitrites, and N-nitroso compounds comes from various sources. Nitrosamines may occur as contaminants in foods, through treatment with nitrate or nitritie, or as a result of food processing. When N-nitrosodimethylamine (NDMA) was found as a contaminant in beer, it was traced to the process of drying malt and hops, which was then altered by the manufacturers so as to reduce the concentrations of NDMA in beer to negligible levels (10,11). Thus far, no dietary nitrosamine has been shown to be a human carcinogen. It is impossible to say how the levels of NDMA previously found in beer are implicated in cancer causation. The amounts of nitrite added to cured meat products have in recent years been reduced (12). Although nitrite itself has not been shown to be carcinogenic, it may react in the stomach to produce various N-nitroso compounds that might be carcinogenic. Some vegetables and fruits naturally contain large amounts of nitrate; however, these foods also contain ascorbic acid, which is an inhibitor of nitrosation. Several geographic epidemiological studies have shown that high levels of nitrate or nitrite in soil and drinking water may be associated with an increased incidence of human stomach and esophageal cancer (13–15). However, these are not among the major cancers in the United States and the incidence of stomach cancer has been decreasing over the last 50 years (16). The possible effects of nitrate or nitrite in foods and water in relation to human carcinogenesis are difficult to assess and evaluate as to their contribution to the total cancer rate. We should, however, proceed cautiously in this regard.

Because chemicals that cause mutations have a higher probability of being initiators of carcinogenesis, much research is currently being carried out on the mutagenic activity found in foods, particularly fried and cooked foods. Many of these mutagens have not yet been adequately tested for carcinogenicity (17). Of those tested, the data are conflicting. However, as mutagens continue to be isolated, they will need to be tested for carcinogenicity in animals. Even if found to cause cancer in animals at specific sites, many factors need consideration before any actions to reduce exposure can be taken.

The state of the evidence, then, suggests that the extent of the carcinogenic effect from exogenous sources is probably weak. Although many substances are tumorigenic in experimental animals and a smaller number carcinogenic for humans, the effects of possible low-dose or low-potency carcinogens, not by themselves sufficient to induce malignancy, are enhanced by significant modifying factors, so that the greater influence of nutritional components on human cancer is not in the area of genotoxic agents, but rather is due to the elements of nutrition acting as epigenetic promoting agents, cocarcinogens, or tumor modifiers. Thus, the overall action of carcinogenesis may depend largely on promoting activity, and it is here that the carcinogenic process may be most susceptible to modification.

The whole area of specific initiating or genotoxic agents in our diet constitutes a field of assumptions that are very difficult to prove at this time with the probable exception of aflatoxin. Specific tumorigenic agents are perhaps present in diets in various parts of the world, but if we overfocus on the elusive genotoxins we may be overlooking a good chance of reducing the occurrence of cancer by modifying the promoting process. It is, after all, not necessary to understand the pathogenesis of cancer and the mechanisms of cancer causation completely to initiate preventive measures based on what is reliably known now. By investigating those factors of our daily diet that bear a significant relationship to the most common cancers, that is, specific nutritional deficiencies and an unbalanced or overloaded metabolic capability from dietary excesses, such as dietary fat, we can achieve a greater impact on cancer prevention.

DIETARY DEFICIENCY FACTORS

Dietary deficiencies, especially when subclinical, are difficult to evaluate. Table 10-1 lists specific dietary components whose deficiencies are suspected to increase the risk of certain types of cancer. The question re-

Table 10.1   Nutritional Deficiencies that Relate to Cancer Risk

Deficient Dietary Component	Related Cancers	Postulated Mechanisms
Vitamin A and its precursors	Lung, esophagus, larynx, bladder	Enhancement of protective cellular mechanisms present in epithelia; metaplasia
Vitamin C	Gastric, esophagus, larynx	Inbhibits in vivo nitrosation reactions
Riboflavin	Upper alimentary tract	Atrophy, hyperkeratosis, hyperplasia of upper alimentary tract cells; effect on mitochondrial respiratory enzymes as a lack of cofactor
Iron	Upper alimentary tract (Plummer-Vinson syndrome), gastric	Indirect effects resulting from iron deficiency
Iodine	Follicular carcinoma of thyroid; breast	Affects hormone secretions? Increases estrogen receptors in breast?
Selenium	Colon, breast	Functions as part of the enzyme glutathione peroxidase; interaction with heavy metals?
Fiber	Colon	Dilution and binding of carcinogens and promoters

mains to what extent recommendations are in order to the public or to the food industry to overcome these deficiencies. The food industry has, for instance, introduced iodized salt, which led to a decline of goiter and thyroid cancer, and in Sweden, flour was fortified with iron and B vitamins—steps that led to a reduction of Plummer-Vinson disease as well as of related cancers of the upper alimentary tract (18, 19).

It has been suggested that the high incidence of esophageal cancer in certain parts of Iran and China is related to dietary deficiencies, specifically diets low in fresh fruits and vegetables, and hence to low estimated intakes of vitamin A, vitamin C, and riboflavin (20,21). Upper alimentary tract cancers in the Western world correlate with a promoting and/or cocarcinogenic effect of alcohol with tobacco (22,23). Alcohol consumption as an enhancer may act through associated micronutrient deficiencies in vitamin A, riboflavin, iron, and possibly also minerals such as zinc. The exact role of each of these is difficult to determine, since usually deficiencies in specific nutrients are interrelated (24).

Van Rensburg (25) has also suggested that dietary nutritional deficiencies, such as zinc, magnesium, nicotinic acid, and possibly riboflavin, in populations at high risk for esophageal cancer may also occur in alcohol abusers and might increase the susceptibility of the esophageal epithelium to neoplastic transformation.

The deficiency of iron and riboflavin found in alcoholism and Plummer-Vinson syndrome enhances the already present risk of cancers of the upper alimentary tract posed by these diseases by increasing the chances of maglinant transformation of epithelial cells. The roles of iron and riboflavin in cellular oxidation may be implicated. Wynder and Klein (26) found experimentally that riboflavin deficiency resulted in atrophy and then hyperkeratosis of the upper alimentary tract in mice, as well as in the skin of mice, where the riboflavin deficiency was also followed by hyperplasia. Chan and Wynder (27) subsequently demonstrated that riboflavin deficient mice developed tumors more rapidly than control mice on a nutritionally adequate diet. We have proposed a hypothesis that nutritional deficiences in riboflavin or iron or both in conjunction with chronic ethanol intake results in accumulation of fatty acyl coenzyme A esters that inhibit mitochondrial adenine nucleotide translocation, resulting in loss of ATP formation which must then be made up by increased glycolysis. The enhanced formation of NADPH would increase the rates of metabolic activation of procarcinogens by the microsomal mixed function oxidase system in the hyperplastic cell. This creates an intracellular environment for enhanced conversion to the neoplastic state (23, 28).

Vitamin A deficiency may be involved in epithelial neoplasia through an adverse effect on mucous-producing epithelium such as in the lung. Several epidemiologic studies seem to show that a high intake of foods rich in vitamin A or its precursors may have a protective effect against lung cancer (29). Vitamin A intake levels were negatively associated with lung cancer incidence at all levels of cigarette smoking in one study (30), and high intakes of sources of vitamin A reduced the risk for lung cancer associated with cigarette smoking in another study (31). Shekelle and co-workers (32) showed a similar effect of β-carotene on lung cancer at all smoking levels.

Vitamin C deficiency or low seasonal intakes have been associated with gastric cancer (33) and may be due to vitamin C inhibition of nitrosation and prevention of the formation of carcinogenic N-nitroso compounds (34).

The available evidence from both experimental and epidemiologic studies strongly indicates that nutritional deficiencies of the types described are of etiologic significance in the development of some cancers. Evidence of a relationship to nutritional deficiencies has most often been made for esophageal cancer (25), and has been less well documented for gastric cancer (35).

A difficulty in delineating the role of nutritional deficiencies in cancer is due to their being largely subclinical and difficult to determine by nutritional surveys, although Graham (36) has obtained some good leads in this manner. Nutritional deficiencies are, of course, often interlinked, and biochemical studies of blood (serum) and more pertinently of tissues are usually not done. The science of biochemical epidemiology, and especially the enzyme chemist, can contribute significantly to this issue. In fact, observations made by the various disciplines can contribute to better hypotheses that then can be further investigated through an interdisciplinary approach, extending our knowledge and leading us toward better recommendations for prevention.

The final proof of the role of micronutrients in cancer etiology is likely to come from intervention studies using chemo-prevention, that is, the use of natural or synthetic agents to prevent, inhibit, or reverse one or more of the states of carcinogenesis. Researchers in the field of chemical carcinogenesis have identified some substances, such as vitamine C and E, β-carotene, antabuse, selenium, and the food preservative antioxidants butylated hydroxytoluene (BHT) and butylated hyroxyanisole (BHA), among others, that can inhibit tumor formation in animals (37). Some epidemiologic studies seemed to find a decreased risk of colon cancer associated with eating certain cruciferous vegetables (38, 39), paralleling the finding in animals. Studies in humans on the effects of metabolism of certain drugs indicated that subjects eating diets rich in vegetables such as Brussels sprouts and cabbage metabolized antipyrine and phenacetin more rapidly than control subjects (40). The oxidative metabolism of these compounds may be similar to that of some carcinogens and seems to be influenced by dietary factors.

Fiber, of course, can also be considered as a chemopreventive because it has established effects on stool bulk and consistency and lower intestinal motility. A higher fiber consumption prevents and relieves constipation and diverticular disease and acts as a protective factor in the etiology of large bowel cancer (41).

NUTRITIONAL EXCESSES—METABOLIC OVERLOAD

It is our view that overnutrition resulting in metabolic overload has a significant effect on human carcinogenesis. Overnutrition acts largely as a tumor modifier on the basis of a variety of mechanisms (Table 10-2). The effects of total caloric intake have been difficult to assess with respect to the risk of cancer, because of the variables resulting from the composition of the diet. Thus, it is difficult to evaluate total intake versus specific macronutrient intake. Any observed effects may be due to a specific nutrient. Of course, overweight persons would benefit in any case by decreasing their total caloric intake, including fat calories. Since the contribution of proteins to total calories is nearly constant in most populations, though its sources may vary, the effect of overnutrition must relate principally to the fat/carbohydrate ratio.

When the intake of pickled, salted, and smoked foods is high and the intake of fresh fruits and vegetables is low, the incidence of gastric cancer is high (33,34). If the intake of fat is high, both in terms of saturated and unsaturated fats, a variety of cancers have high prevalence—notably breast, colon, and prostrate, but also pancreas, bladder, ovary, and endometrium (42).

In applying the criteria for judgment outlined by the First Surgeon General's Report on Smoking and Health (3), for making critical ap-

Table 10.2   Current Concepts on Colon Cancer Causation and Development[a]

Risk factors		
Diets high in fat, cholesterol, fried foods, and low in fiber and in green-yellow vegetables		
Postulated mechanisms		
High fat	High cholesterol biosynthesis	High gut bile acid levels
	High dietary cholesterol	
Low fiber (lack of bulk)	High concentration of gut bile acids (low dilution through lack of bulk)	
High bile acid concentration	Promoting effect in colon carcinogenesis	
Mechansims under study		
Fried food	Mutagens	Colon carcinogens?
Role of micronutrients (vitamins and minerals) and different types of fiber in production and metabolism of carcinogens, bile acids, promoters?		
Mechanisms of promotion?		

[a]Reproduced and reprinted with permission from (110).

praisals of data, interpreting and formulating conclusions, we concur with the conclusion of the National Academy of Sciences Committee that the association of fat to the etiology of cancer of the breast and colon is "most suggestive of a causal relationship."

This concept is supported by the following observations:

1. Epidemiological studies of the widely varying international cancer incidence and mortality rates correlated with intake of specific dietary components in different countries worldwide, show that significantly positive correlations exist between total fat disappearance data and breast and colon cancer rates (43–46). The highest incidence of these cancers occurs in the Western world and the low-risk areas are found in Japan and Asia.

2. The risk of colon and breast cancers closely parallels the economic development of countries, showing a rising incidence with increased Westernization of diet, specifically a higher fat intake (42, 47, 48).

3. The incidence and mortality rates shift as migrants move from areas of low risk, such as Japan, to areas of higher risk, such as the United States, so that the migrants' rates increase and become those of the new area of residence as they adopt new food habits (49–53). The rate of colon cancer shows a rise in the first generation, and the breast cancer rate rises in the second generation of Japanese migrants to the United States.

4. Students of special population groups support the association between high fat diets and breast cancer (54–59), as well as colon cancer, where such studies have also suggested the role of certain fibers as protective agents (60–64).

5. Case/control studies have provided suggestive evidence that patients with breast cancer or with colon cancer (53, 65, 66) consume more fat than controls. Because of the difficulty in obtaining proper long-term nutritional histories, such data need careful evaluation (36, 67).

6. Time trends in the United States for colon and breast cancer show only a small increase in incidence over several decades, indicating that the causes and modifiers of these cancers have been in the environment for a long time (68–71).

7. Experimental studies in animal models by a variety of carcinogens differing in metabolic activation mechanisms nonetheless show repeatedly and reproducibly that animals fed a high-fat diet (20%, equivalent to the 40% of calories in the Western diet) have a greater incidence of colon and mammary tumors than animals fed a low-fat diet (5%, equivalent to the 10% of calories of fat in a low-risk population) (42, 72, 73). The fat effect seems to appear at the promotion stage of carcinogenesis (44, 72, 74). Such studies have provided substantial leads to mechanisms whereby fat exerts its effects.

8. Metabolic (biochemical) epidemiologic studies investigating fecal constituents of populations with diverse dietary habits and those investigating breast secretions are providing new observations generally consistent with the descriptive epidemiological data (42, 61, 75–79).

For both cancers, then, there is a close association in populations with a high total fat intake. The difference in increase of colon and breast cancers as a function of migrant generation may relate to exposure to initiating genotoxic carcinogens during periods of active tissue and cell proliferation and DNA synthesis that take place at the time of puberty during breast development (80). The neoplastic growth and development of the initiated cell may occur later in life under conditions that promote such changes, namely, the effects of a high-fat diet. This is borne out by laboratory animal studies which indicated that the effect of high fat intake is exerted primarily on the postinitiation (promotional) phase of breast carcinogenesis (72, 74).

BREAST CANCER

Experiments designed to mimic the human environment with respect to breast cancer in animal models have yielded a reliable data base. Experiments were undertaken using intakes of high levels of saturated or unsaturated fats, equivalent to those consumed by Western people (typically 20% by weight or 40% by calories). These studies have uniformly demonstrated an increased incidence and multiplicity of mammary gland cancer in rats or mice previously given a suitable carcinogen. In the case of mice inoculated with the mammary tumor virus, no carcinogen was required (42). The reference level of fat in most of these cases was 5% in the diet, or 10% of calories, equivalent to the fat intake in a low risk population such as the Japanese during the 1950s (47, 81). Where a fat level of 0.5% in the diet was used, basically similar results were obtained, although the levels of essential fatty acids, and thus of overall nutritional status, may have been limiting (44). With a 5% fat level, female rats given a carcinogen had a somewhat lower total tumor burden of breast cancer when the fat was saturated than when it was unsaturated. Administration of a combination of a small amount (3%) of unsaturated oil plus saturated fat gave an even higher tumor burden of breast cancer in rats than the equivalent amount of oil or fat alone (82).

Specific mechanisms whereby fat exerts its effects in the development of breast cancer remain to be elucidated. Evidence suggests that the fat effect may be mediated by alterations in host endocrine systems, prostaglandin levels, or hormone receptor levels (83, 84). Attention has focused on the hormone prolactin because there is experimental evidence which indicates that prolactin and estrogen may be the most essential to growth and development of rodent mammary tumors (85–87).

Because prolactin is a known tumor promoter in experimental breast cancer (88), changes in prolactin secretion patterns may underlie the association between fat consumption and breast cancer risk demonstrated by epidemiologic analysis. Chan and Cohen (89) have demonstrated in rats that high-fat diets increase serum prolactin concentrations. Dietary fats increased the nocturnal surge of prolactin in the serum of women volunteers on a standard high-fat Western diet (90), whereas healthy postmenopausal vegetarian women exhibited decreased plasma prolactin levels compared to age-matched nonvegetarian women (79). Such human studies support the animal data. However, the situation is much more complex and we are probably dealing with nutrition controlling endocrine balances, involving hormones from pituitary, thyroid, adrenals, fat cells, bacterial flora, and gonads (especially in premenopausal women).

As an alternative approach, it has been proposed that rather than looking in the serum or urine, examination of breast duct fluid, the secretion of which is less common among Japanese and Chinese women than among white women, may yield better information (76, 91, 92) because the ductal fluid is in intimate contact with the alveolar ductal cells of mammary glands where most breast tumors originate and has been shown to contain mutagenic substances (93). Comparing the contents of duct fluids from women in the United States (high risk), Finland (intermediate risk), and Japan (low risk) may therefore provide insight into the etiologic factors of breast cancer. Petrakis and his co-workers (94) have suggested that cholesterol epoxides identified in breast secretion might have tumorigenic activity. The cellular material in the breast aspirates of Western women, which is greater than that in Japanese women (95, 96), may relate to a hyperplastic effect of their breast secretions on ductal epithelium, leading to exfoliation of epithelial cells (97). Differences in cytological material present in breast fluid from populations at differing risk for breast cancer may reflect the integrity of the ductal epithelium of the breast in Western and Japanese women that might bear on the relative differences in breast cancer risk (98). In a study of breast fluid from Finnish women (76), hormone analyses centered on prolactin and estrogens, which were found in higher concentrations in breast fluid of healthy women than in their serum. In both Western and Japanese women, the hormone concentrations of estrogens and prolactins are higher in the breast secretions than in the serum. The function of the hormones present in the ductal fluid is not known.

We suggest that a high intake of dietary fat affects the lipid contents of breast secretions, and may further alter the concentration of hormones, hormone receptors, or both.

Colon Cancer

Human studies investigating fecal constitutents of populations with diverse dietary habits indicate that individuals on a high-fat diet have a higher level of fecal secondary bile acids and gut microbial activity as measured by certain bacterial enzymes (42, 78). The metabolic epidemiologic data demonstrate a correlation between fecal bile acid metabolites and the risk for colon cancer in diverse populations (42, 99). Such studies have also shown that patients with colon cancer or with adenomatous polyps have a higher concentration of these metabolites in their feces than control patients (100). Endogenously, a high-fat diet enhances the biliary secretion of bile acids and modifies activity of gut microflora, increasing the formation of secondary bile acids in the colon (101, 102). Since the fractional reabsorption of bile acids in terminal ileum is constant, dietary fat directly affects total fecal bile acid concentrations in the large intestine and fecal output. Certain bile acids promote colon cancer in rats initiated with direct-acting carcinogens, such as MNNG, increasing the total number of tumors in both conventional and germfree rats (103). A high intake of certain dietary fibers, such as wheat bran and whole grain cereals, which are rich in cellulose and hemicellulose, leads to an increased stool bulk, thereby diluting the colonic concentration of certain secondary bile acids that accompany high levels of fat intake (78, 104). High fecal bulk decreases the concentration of fecal secondary bile acids but does not lower the daily output of these putative promoting compounds in both humans and rats on a high intake of dietary fat (104). Uncertainties in fiber studies in experimental systems may be due to the varying capacities of such fibers not only to increase stool bulk, but also to bind several of these compounds (41). In addition, the carcinogen load also affects the fiber capacity; the promoting stimulus is more readily visualized when the carcinogen action is only moderate. Any protective effect on promotion due to dilution by fiber increasing stool bulk is seen only when the effect of the carcinogen is not overwhelming. The situation in man most likely involves low carcinogen loads because increased stool bulk due to fiber intake, as exemplified in Finland (105) and in Mormon populations (106), strikingly becomes a protective effect even in people basically on a high-fat dietary regimen. This "chemopreventive" system also demonstrates that lowering the concentration of promoting bile acids by one-third to two-thirds is most effective in reducing colon cancer risk. This dose-response phenomenon for promoters requires further extension to other situations.

Mechanisms of Action

The mechanisms through which dietary fat exerts its tumor-promoting effects in the nutritionally linked cancers are not fully documented but probably can be categorized as those involving direct effects of fat on tumor development and those involving indirect effects on host metabolism. Direct effects relate to changes in the lipid content of the cell membrane or membrane-bound receptors and the synthesis of prostaglandins. Indirect mechanisms involve changes in the immune system, enhanced activity of mixed function oxidase systems in carcinogen production and metabolism, or steroid metabolism, alterations in fecal flora and bile acid metabolism, and alterations in the endocrine milieu of the host. Thus, a role of dietary fat in the promotion, though probably not in the initiation, of cancer at various sites is biologically plausible. We thus have a full circle of pieces of evidence.

If we reason from an evolutionary point of view, it would seem evident that our metabolic capacities have not been prepared for our fat overload, leading to cardiovascular disease when cholesterol is dispersed in the arterial walls, to colon cancer as we increase the amount of bile acids in the stool, and to breast cancer as we influence the hormonal milieu and its lipid nature within the breast. This effect is not so much on the basis of obesity, which has its major effects on cancer of the endometrium and the gallbladder, but largely through excesses of fat leading to an overload of specific metabolic pathways that adversely affect tissues and cells. Our ideas call for optimal rather than normal values for serum cholesterol as related to cardiovascular disease (107) and for bile acid concentrations in the stool as they relate to colon cancer (108). Cancer, after all, can result if we excessively expose ourselves to initiating genotoxic agents or even more so to promoting epigenetic agents. Why should we be surprised, why should it not be logical, that excesses of specific chemical or physical agents can be injurious to our cells and tissues, and thus to our bodies?

DIETARY RECOMMENDATIONS

The German philosopher Kant noted that often in life we have to make decisions on the basis of knowledge sufficient for action but insufficient to satisfy the intellect. As public health authorities we need to recognize that by making no decision we have left a status quo which in our case would be the continuance of the incidence of and mortality from diseases that are associated with dietary factors. Thus, such a course of inaction may already have contributed to the prevalence of diseases, such as colon, breast, and prostate cancers, as well as coronary heart disease, or to the future incidence of these diseases in some areas of the world, previously largely spared, such as Japan and the Middle East, where Western dietary habits are being increasingly adopted. A distinguished jurist, Judge D. Bazelon (109), has reached similar conclusions in relation to the role of the judiciary in health matters.

Hippocrates stated many centuries ago that a therapeutic recommendation should, above all, do no harm. Clearly, the recommendations we make for dietary modifications are consistent with the philosophy found in the sayings of both Kant and Hippocrates. It is time to make a dietary recommendation to the public and to food producers on the basis of prudence based upon the best available medical and scientific evidence, in the hope of reducing the incidence not merely of certain types of cancer but also of other diseases, including cardiovascular diseases and adult-onset diabetes—all related to nutritional excesses.

The National Academy of Sciences' Committee has proposed dietary recommendations, as did the National Cancer Institute, the National Heart, Lung, and Blood Institute, the American Cancer Society, and the American Heart Association. Our recommendations (Table 10-3) are more specific in numbers and suggest a lower intake, particularly of fat to 20–25%, than the other recommendations. The evidence, however, suggests that when it comes to fat, less is better than more, especially for a sedentary population. The importance of these nutritional recommendations relates not only to the limits of intake of macronutrients (fat and simple carbohydrates), and the optimal levels for others (fibers, complex carbohydrates, and vegetable proteins), but also to the area of micronutrients, although here we cannot give specific levels. We should consume micronutrients not as supplements, though evidence for this may be forthcoming in the future, but principally by increasing the use of foods wherein they are mainly contained, such as green and yellow

Table 10.3 American Health Foundation Food Plan[a]

Contents	1000 Calories per Day		1500 Calories per Day		2000 Calories per Day	
	%	Calories	%	Calories	%	Calories
Protein (including) vegetable protein)	12	120	12	180	12	240
Fat	20–25	200	20–25	300–375	20–25	400–500
Saturated fat	7–8	70	7–8	100–125	7–8	140–160
Monounsaturated fat	7–8	70	7–8	100–125	7–8	140–160
Polyunsaturated fat	7–8	70	7–8	100–125	7–8	140–160
Carbohydrate (mostly complex carbohydrate)	68	680	63–68	945–1020	63–68	1260–1360
Other dietary components						
Dietary fiber	35 g/day		35 g/day		35 g/day	
Salt	3–5 g/d		3–5 g/day		3–5 g/day	
Cholesterol	200 mg/day		200 mg/day		200 mg/day	

[a]Adapted from (111). Because of rounding off, figures may not add up to 100%.

vegetables. The nutrients zinc and vitamin B_{12} are usually derived from animal protein products. Substantial amounts of zinc can be obtained from whole-grain products, brewer's yeast, wheat bran, and wheat germ, but vitamin B_{12} is found almost only in animal protein. Liver is the best source, and a low-fat diet would probably still include enough B_{12} from fish, meats, and dairy products, whereas complete vegetarians might have to take supplements. Overconsumption of alcohol may cause a B_{12} deficiency.

The prudent diet, or rather the day-by-day eating regimen, prescribes what we should eat more of, and what we should eat less of. This should involve lifelong habits started in infancy and should provide us with optimal physical and mental well-being. Prudence as far as the impact on nutrition is concerned is a lifelong experience. The medical profession has been remiss in not recognizing what popular thinking has long held to be self-evident; that is, "we are what we eat." This truism applies to the life of each cell as well as it does to the whole organism. As science recognizes this more fully, we shall advance toward preventing what we know are nutrition-related diseases.

No doubt national and international efforts in the next decade will develop more sound information through active research programs on the mechanisms of action of specific macro- and micronutrients, of select food additives such as synthetic and natural antioxidants, and of the mode of cooking, in causing, promoting, or inhibiting each kind of nutritionally linked cancer. This broad multidisciplinary approach to the multifactorial complex causes of the major kinds of cancer should yield an even firmer base of public action (Figure 10-1). In the meantime, the research of the last 15 years or longer has led us to the sound data base that is desirable for the beginning of public health action. This involves a strategy to reduce total fat intake and increase the consumption of complex carbohydrates and fiber in most of the Western world (Figure 10-2, Table 10-4). Furthermore, these facts suggest that other countries also adopt nutritional habits consonant with the documented findings of research thus far.

The opportunities in this field are considerable for researchers and public health authorities. To achieve the full potential of research and public health action as it relates to nutritional carcinogenesis, it may be useful to consider the development of multidisciplinary nutrition-based

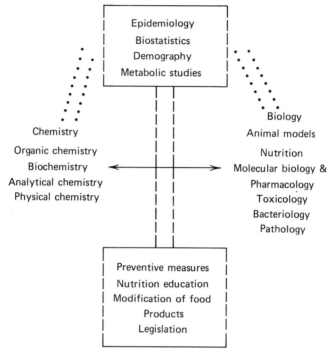

Figure 10-1. Interdisciplinary approach to nutritional carcinogenesis. A working interrelationship of many scientific disciplines is necessary to fully explore the complex question of nutritional carcinogenesis. Such an interdisciplinary approach both provides and utilizes a sound data basis for cancer prevention.

units that because of certain critical mass can accomplish more in these areas than individual scientists or groups working in isolation. We believe that, as we advance the knowledge of nutritional causes of carcinogenesis through such or similar units, we may more readily overcome limitations that exist in nutritional research in general and nutritional carcinogenesis efforts in particular. At the same time, the creation of such units would accelerate the fulfillment of the opportunities that exist in basic research and in preventive applications in the broad area of nutrition as they relate to cancer and to disease in general.

Our resolve can have a major impact on the incidence of cancer and other chronic diseases.

We wish to thank Ms. Clara Horn for assisting in the preparation of the manuscript.

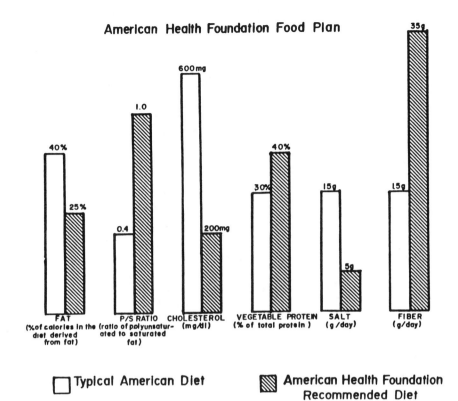

Figure 10-2. American Health Foundation Food Plan. The American Health Foundation recommended diet emphasizes lowering total fat content of our diet by 15% of calories and particularly lowering the saturated fat portion so that the ratio of polyunsaturated to saturated fats is even. A concomitant lowering of cholesterol would result. Protein derived from vegetable products, including breads and cereals, should be increased by eating more legumes and grains that would also increase the fiber content of the diet to recommended levels. Salt intake should be reduced in kind.

Table 10.4   Public Health Implications

A.	Geographic Pathology	Epidemiology
	Low fat, Japan	Low risk for myocardial infarction and colon cancer
	High fat–high fiber, Finland	High risk for myocardial infarction and low risk for colon cancer
	High fat–low fiber, United States	High risk for myocardial infarction and high risk for colon cancer
B.	Public Health Action Lower total fat Increase complex fiber	Prevention of myocardial infarction and colon cancer

REFERENCES

1. National Academy of Sciences National Research Council Committee on Diet, Nutrition, and Cancer, *Diet, Nutrition and Cancer,* Washington, D.C., National Academy Press, 1982.

2. Council for Agricultural Science and Technology (CAST), *Diet, Nutrition, and Cancer: A Critique,* CAST Special Publ. No. 13, Ames, Iowa, 1982.

3. U.S. Dept. Health, Education and Welfare, *Smoking and Health. Rept. of the Advisory Committee to the Surgeon General of the Public Health Service,* U.S. Public Health Svc. Pub. No. 1103, 1964, pp. 19–21; U.S. Dept. Health, Education and Welfare, *Health Consequences of Smoking—Cancer.* A Report of the Surgeon General, Washington, D.C., U.S. Dept. Health and Human Services, DHHS (PHS) 82-50179, 1982.

4. W. T. London, *Human Pathology,* **12,** 1085 (1981).

5. International Agency for Research on Cancer (IARC), *On the Evaluation of Carcinogenic Risk of Chemicals to Man. Some Naturally Occurring Substances,* IARC Monogr. 10, Lyon, France, IARC, 1976.

6. C. A. Linsell and F. G. Peers, in H. Hiatt, J. Watson, and J. Winsten, Eds., *Origins of Human Cancer,* Cold Spring Harbor, N.Y. Cold Spring Harbor Laboratory, 1977, pp. 549–556.

7. L. Stoloff, *J. Assoc. Anal. Chem.,* **63,** 1067 (1980).

8. T. H. Jukes, in *Diet, Nutrition, and Cancer: A Critique,* CAST Special Publ. No. 13, Ames, Iowa, 1982, pp. 79–85.

9. E. V. Jensen, in *Diet, Nutrition, and Cancer: A Critique,* CAST Special Publ. No. 13, Ames, Iowa, 1982, pp. 41–43.

10. R. Preussmann, B. Spiegelhalder, and G. Eisenbrand, in R. A. Scanlan and S. R. Tannenbaum, Eds., *N-Nitroso Compounds,* ACS Symposium Series 174, Washington, D.C., American Chemical Society, 1981, p. 217.

11. M. M. Mangino and R. A. Scanlan, in R. A. Scanlan and S. R. Tannenbaum, Eds., *N-Nitroso Compounds,* ACS Symposium Series 174, Washington, D.C., American Chemical Society, 1981, p. 229.

12. E. F. Binkerd and O. E. Kolari, *Food Cosmet. Toxicol.,* **13,** 655 (1975).

13. R. Armijo, A. Gonzalez, M. Orellana, A. H. Coulson, J. W. Sayre, and R. Detels, *Int. J. Epidemiol.,* **10,** 57 (1981).

14. P. Correa, W. Haenszel, C. Cuello, S. Tannenbaum, and M. Archer, *Lancet,* **2,** 1975.

15. C. Cuello, P. Correa, W. Haenszel, G. Gordillo, C. Brown, M. Archer, and S. Tannenbaum, *J. Natl. Cancer Inst.,* **57,** 1015 (1976).

16. American Cancer Society, *1983 Cancer Facts and Figures,* New York, American Cancer Society, 1983.

17. T. Sugimura, T. Kawachi, M. Nagao, T. Yahagi, in G. R. Newell and M. N. Ellison, Eds., *Nutrition and Cancer: Etiology and Treatment,* New York, Raven, 1981, p. 59.

18. L. G. Larsson, A. Sandström, and P. Westling, *Cancer Res.,* **35,** 3308 (1975).

19. E. L. Wynder, S. Hultberg, F. Jacobsson, and I. J. Bross, *Cancer,* **10,** 470 (1957).

20. Joint Iran-International Agency for Research on Cancer Study Group, *J. Natl. Cancer Inst.,* **59,** 1127 (1977).

21. P. S. Cook-Mozaffari, F. Azordegan, N. E. Day, et al., *Br. J. Cancer,* **39,** 293 (1979).

22. A. J. McMichael, *Lancet*, **1**, 1244 (1978).

23. G. D. McCoy and E. L. Wynder, *Cancer Res.*, **39**, 2844 (1979).

24. B. Kissin and M. M. Kaley, in B. Kissin and H. Begleiter, Eds., *The Biology of Alcoholism*, Vol. 3, New York-London, Plenum, 1974, pp. 481–511.

25. S. J. van Rensburg, *J. Natl. Cancer Inst.*, **67**, 243 (1981).

26. E. L. Wynder and U. E. Klein, *Cancer*, **18**, 167 (1965).

27. E. L. Wynder and P. C. Chan, *Cancer*, **26**, 1221 (1970).

28. P. C. Chan, T. Okamoto, and E. L. Wynder, *J. Natl. Cancer Inst.*, **48**, 1341 (1972).

29. R. Peto, R. Doll, J. D. Buckley, M. B. Sporn, *Nature (London)*, **290**, 201 (1981).

30. E. Bjelke, *Intl. J. Cancer*, **15**, 561 (1975).

31. R. MacLennan, J. DaCosta, N. E. Day, et al., *Intl. J. Cancer*, **20**, 854 (1977).

32. R. B. Shekelle, M. Lepper, S. Liu, C. Maliza, W. J. Raynor, Jr., A. H. Rossof, O. Paul, A. M. Shryock, and J. Stamler, *Lancet*, **2**, 1185 (1981).

33. J. H. Weisburger, in R. A. Scanlan and S. R. Tannenbaum, Eds., *N-Nitroso Compounds, ACS Symposium Series 174*, Washington, D.C., American Chemical Society, 1981, p. 305.

34. S. S. Mirvish, *J. Toxicol. Environ. Health*, **2**, 1267 (1977).

35. P. Correa, *Cancer*, **50**, 2554 (1982).

36. S. Graham and C. Mettlin, *Am. J. Epidemiol.*, **109**, 1 (1979).

37. L. W. Wattenberg and L. K. T. Lam, in M. S. Zedeck and M. Lipkin, Eds., *Inhibition of Tumor Induction and Development*, New York, Plenum, 1981, p. 1.

38. E. Bjelke, *Thesis, University of Minnesota*, University Microfilms Ann Arbor (1973).

39. S. Graham, *Banbury Rept.*, **7**, (1981).

40. A. H. Conney, M. K. Buening, E. J. Pantuck, C. B. Pantuck, J. G. Fortner, K. E. Anderson, and A. Kappas, in *Environmental Chemicals, Enzyme Function and Human Disease*, Ciba Foundation Symposium 76 (new series), Amsterdam, Excerpta Medica, 1980, p. 147.

41. R. M. Kay, *J. Lipid Res.*, **23**, 221 (1982).

42. B. S. Reddy, L. A. Cohen, G. D. McCoy, P. Hill, J. H. Weisburger, and E. L. Wynder, *Adv. Cancer Res.*, **32**, 237 (1980).

43. B. Armstrong and R. Doll, *Int. J. Cancer*, **15**, 617 (1975).

44. K. K. Carroll, *Cancer Res.*, **35**, 3374 (1975).

45. G. E. Gray, M. C. Pike, B. E. Henderson, *Br. J. Cancer*, **39**, 1 (1979).

46. A. B. Miller, *Cancer*, **39**, 2704 (1977).

47. T. Hirayama, *Nutrit. Cancer*, **1**, 67 (1979).

48. E. L. Wynder and T. Hirayama, *Prev. Med.*, **6**, 567 (1977)

49. P. Buell, *J. Natl. Cancer Inst.*, **51**, 1479 (1973).

50. B. McMahon, P. Cole, and J. Brown, *J. Natl. Cancer Inst.*, **50**, 21 (1973).

51. J. F. Fraumeni, Jr., Ed., *Persons at High Risk of Cancer*, New York, Academic, 1975.

52. D. Schottenfeld and J. F. Fraumeni, Jr., *Cancer Epidemiology and Prevention*, Phila., Saunders, 1982.

53. J. E. Dunn, *Natl. Cancer Inst. Monogr.*, **47**, 157 (1977).

54. R. L. Phillips, *Cancer Res.*, **35**, 3513 (1975).

55. R. L. Phillips, J. W. Kuzma, W. L. Beeson, and T. Lotz, *Am. J. Epidemiol.*, **112**, 296 (1980).

56. A. Nomura, G. N. Stemmermann, G. G. Rhoads, and G. A. Glober, *Hawaii Med. J.*, **34**, 309 (1973).

57. D. M. Ingram, *Nutr. Cancer*, **3**, 75 (1982).

58. E. L. Wynder, F. A. MacCornack, S. D. Stellman, *Cancer*, **41**, 2341 (1978).

59. F. de Waard, J. P. Cornelis, K. Aoki, M. Yoshida, *Cancer*, **40**, 1269 (1977).

60. W. Haenszel, J. W. Berg, M. Segi, M. Kurihara, F. B. Locke, *J. Natl. Cancer Inst.*, **51**, 1765 (1973).

61. B. S. Reddy, A. Hedges, K. Laakso, and E. L. Wynder, *Cancer*, **42**, 2832 (1978).

62. J. L. Lyon, J. W. Gardner, and D. W. West, *Banbury Rept.*, **4**, 3 (1980).

63. A. J. McMichael, M. G. McCall, J. M. Hartshorne, and T. L. Woodings, *Int. J. Cancer*, **35**, 431 (1980).

64. D. P. Burkitt, in S. J. Winawer, D. Schottenfeld, and P. Sherlock, Eds., *Progress in Cancer Research and Therapy*, Vol. 13, New York, Raven, 1980, p. 13.

65. A. B. Miller, A. Kelly, N. W. Choi, V. Matthews, R. W. Morgan, L. Munan, J. D. Burch, J. Feather, G. R. Howe, and M. Jain, *Am. J. Epid.*, **107**, 499 (1978).

66. M. Jain, G. M. Cooke, F. G. Davis, M. G. Grace, G. R. Howe, and A. B. Miller, *Int. J. Cancer*, **26**, 757 (1980).

67. A. E. Harper and M. Z. Nichaman, *Am. J. Clin. Nutr.*, **35**, 1241 (1982).

68. E. Silverberg, *Ca-A Cancer J. Clinicians*, **31**, 13 (1981).

69. S. S. Devesa and D. T. Silverman, *J. Environ. Pathol. Toxicol.*, **3**, 127 (1980).

70. S. S. Devesa and D. T. Silverman, *J. Natl. Cancer Inst.*, **60**, 545 (1978).

71. S. J. Cutler and J. L. Young, *Natl. Cancer Inst. Monogr.*, **41**, 1 (1975).

72. K. Carroll, *J. Environ. Path. Toxicol.*, **3**(4), 253 (1980).

73. G. J. Hopkins and C. E. West, *Life Sci.*, **19**, 1103 (1976).

74. A. W. Bull, B. K. Soullier, P. S. Wilson, M. T. Hayden, and N. D. Nigro, *Cancer Res.*, **39**, 4956 (1979).

75. I. A. Macdonald, G. R. Webb, and D. C. Mahoney, *Am. J. Clin. Nutr.*, **32**, S233 (1978).

76. E. L. Wynder, P. Hill, K. Laakso, R. Littner, and K. Kettunen, *Cancer*, **47**, 1444 (1981).

77. N. L. Petrakis, V. L. Ernster, S. T. Sacks, E. B. King, R. J. Schweltzer, T. K. Hunt, and M. D. King, *J. Natl. Cancer Inst.*, **67**, 277 (1981).

78. M. Hill, R. McLennan, K. Newcombe, *Lancet*, **1**, 436 (1979).

79. B. K. Armstrong, *Nutr. Cancer*, **1**, 38 (1979).

80. A. B. Miller and R. D. Bulbrook, *N. Engl. J. Med.*, **303**, 1246 (1980).

81. T. Oiso, *Cancer Res.*, **35**, 3254 (1975).

82. K. K. Carroll, *Cancer Res.*, **41**, 3695 (1981).

83. M. M. King, D. M. Bailey, D. D. Gibson, J. V. Pitha, and P. B. McCay, *J. Natl. Cancer Inst.*, **63**, 657 (1979).

84. L. A. Cohen, *Cancer Res.*, **41**, 3808 (1981).

85. T. L. Dao, *Prog. Exp. Tumor Res.*, **11**, 235 (1969).

86. O. H. Pearson, O. Llerena, L. Llerena, A. Molina, and T. Butler, *Trans. Assoc. Am. Physicians,* **82,** 225 (1969).

87. J. Furth, in F. Becker, Ed., *Cancer, A Comprehensive Treatise,* Vol. 1 (2nd ed.), New York, Plenum, 1982, p. 75.

88. P. C. Chan and L. A. Cohen, *J. Natl. Cancer Inst.,* **52,** 25 (1974).

89. C. W. Welsch and H. Nagasawa, *Cancer Res.,* **37,** 951 (1977).

90. P. Hill and E. L. Wynder, *Lancet,* **2,** 806 (1976).

91. N. L. Petrakis, L. Mason, R. Lee, B. Sugimoto, S. Pawson, and F. Catchpol, *J. Natl. Cancer Inst.,* **54,** 829 (1975).

92. S. R. Wellings, *Path. Res. Pract.,* **166,** 515 (1980).

93. N. L. Petrakis, C. A. Maack, R. E. Lee, and M. Lyon, *Cancer Res.,* **40,** 188 (1980).

94. N. L. Petrakis, L. D. Gruenke, and J. D. Craig, *Cancer Res.,* **41,** 2563, 1981.

95. T. Hirayama, personal communication, 1982.

96. American Health Foundation, unpublished data, 1982.

97. N. L. Petrakis, *Environ. Health Perspect.,* **42,** 97 (1981).

98. G. C. Buehring, *Cancer,* **43,** 1788 (1979).

99. B. S. Reddy and E. L. Wynder, *J. Natl. Cancer Inst.,* **50,** 1437 (1973).

100. B. S. Reddy and E. L. Wynder, *Cancer,* **39,** 2533 (1977).

101. B. R. Goldin and S. L. Gorbach, *J. Natl. Cancer Inst.,* **57,** 371 (1976).

102. B. S. Reddy, S. Mangat, J. H. Weisburger, and E. L. Wynder, *Cancer Res.,* **37,** 3533 (1977).

103. B. S. Reddy, K. Watanabe, J. H. Weisburger, and E. L. Wynder, *Cancer Res.,* **37,** 3238 (1977).

104. B. S. Reddy, *Adv. Nutr. Res.,* **2,** 199 (1979).

105. IARC Microecology Group, *Lancet,* **2,** 207 (1977).

106. J. L. Lyon, J. W. Gardner, and D. W. West, *Banbury Report,* **4,** 3 (1980).

107. E. L. Wynder, Ed., *Prev. Med.,* **8,** 609 (1979).

108. E. L. Wynder, R. M. Kay, B. S. Reddy, C. Horn, and J. H. Weisburger, in H. Autrup and C. Harris, Eds., *Human Carcinogenesis,* New York, Academic, 1983, in press.

109. D. L. Bazelon, *Science,* **211,** 792 (1981).

110. J. H. Weisburger, and C. Horn, *Bull. N.Y. Acad. Med.,* **58,** 296 (1982).

111. E. L. Wynder, S. Hertzberg, and E. Parker, eds., *The Book of Health,* New York, Franklin Watts, 1981, p. 32.

Index

Aging:
  effects of nutrition on, 141–142,
      156–158
  nutritional requirements during,
      146–164
  physiological changes during, 142–145
  theories of, 140–141
Alzheimer's disease, 110
Amino acids, 56, 58, 65, 105, 109, 141,
      149
  isoleucine, 105–106
  leucine, 105–106
  phenylalanine, 105
  tryptophan, 103–108, 141
  tyrosine, 103–105, 107–110
  valine, 105–106
Arsenic, 38

Beriberi, 3, 8
Boron, 38

Cadmium, 37, 44
Calcium, 132
  metabolism in aging, 151–154, 161
Cancer:
  breast, 172, 179–183
  colon, 155–156, 172, 179–181, 183–184
  effect of nutrition on, 171–193
  esophagus, 174, 176
  lung, 177
  stomach, 174
  see also Carcinogens
Carbohydrate, 1–2, 4, 51, 103, 107, 109
  craving for, 107
  metabolism of, 8, 91–93

Carcinogens, 172–175
Choline, 103–104, 106, 110
Chromium, 37, 41–42
  deficiency, 42
  dietary sources of, 42
Cobalt, 37
  deficiency, 12
Copper, 11, 37, 41
  deficiency, 41
  influences on bioavailability of, 41
Cytochrome P-450, 23–33

Energy metabolism, 1–2, 87
  in aged, 163
  basal metabolic rate, 88–90, 93–94
  exercise metabolic rate, 98
  metabolic costs of pregnancy, 159–161

Fat, 1–2, 4, 63–64, 91, 95, 143, 172, 189
  increase with aging, 143
  role in carcinogenesis, 175, 178–183
Fetal growth, 48–68
Fetal parasitism, 48, 51
Fiber, 154–156, 175, 183–184, 189
Fluorine, 12, 37

Hemoglobin, 10–11
  role in oxygen transport, 10

Insulin, 92–93, 106
Iodine, 10–12, 37, 175
Iron, 10, 12, 37
  bioavailability of, 39–40, 161, 175–176
  chelators of, 27
  deficiency, 39–40, 161 175–176

Lead, 37
 toxicity of, 37, 43

Magnesium, 8
Malnutrition:
 assessment of consequences of, 113–132
 as cause of immunodeficiency, 16,
  115–117
 and developing brain, 71–79
 diagnosis of, 113
 effect on hepatic secretory proteins,
  114–115
 effect on skeletal muscle function,
  117–130
 recovery from, 82–85
 results of muscle biopsy in, 130–132
Manganese, 11, 37
Maternal-fetal exchange, 56–59
Metabolic rate:
 fetal, 49
 maternal, 49
Methylmercury, 37, 44
Molybdenum, 12, 37

Nickel, 38
Nitrogen, 1, 113, 118, 128, 130–131
 balance studies, 61, 149–150
 retention, 117
Neurotransmitters:
 acetylcholine, 103–104, 109
 catecholamine, 103–104, 108–109
 dopamine, 108
 effects of foods on, 103–111
 lecithin, 106
 norepinephrine, 96, 108–109
 serotonin, 103–104, 106–107
 sphingomyelin, 106
Nutrition:
 and brain evelopment, 71–85
 effects of food restriction, 50–53
 effects on human growth and
  development, 12–14, 47, 50, 79–82
 food intake in elderly, 158–162
 and immunity, 16
 maternal weight gain, 61–62
 and pregnancy, 14–16, 47–68
 role in aging, 138, 141–142, 144
 role in malignant disease, 117, 171–189
 total parenteral, 118

Obesity, 107
 energy expenditure in, 93–96
 genetic, 95
 thermogenesis in, 87–99
Osteoporosis, 153–154

Parkinson's disease, 110–111
Pellagra, 3, 8–9
Potassium, 8, 113, 119, 128, 130, 132, 141
Protein, 1–2, 4, 51, 72, 77, 91, 103,
  106–107, 109, 118, 128, 114
 hepatic secretory proteins, 113–115
 needs of the aging, 149–151, 161,
  163–164
 needs of pregnant women, 60–61

Rickets, 3, 7–8

Scurvy, 3, 5
Selenium, 37
 deficiency, 42–43, 175, 177
Semistarvation, 2
Sodium, 119, 132

Thermic effect of food, 87, 90–93
 during exercise, 96–99
Trace metals, 37
 in human nutrition, 37–44
 interactions of, 43–44

Vitamin A, 6–7, 161, 176–177
 carotene and xanthophyll as sources of,
  6
 deficiency, 3, 6, 39, 116, 175
Vitamin B, 5–6
 biotin, 9
 folic acid, 9, 161
 nicotinic acid, 9
 pantothenic acid, 9
 pyridoxine, 9
 riboflavin, 9, 161, 175–176
 thiamin, 8, 161
 Vitamin B_{12}, 9, 12, 187
Vitamin C, 5, 6, 173, 176
 deficiency, 5–6, 33, 175
 and drug metabolism 21–34

discovery of, 5
    synthesis of, 6
Vitamin D, 7–8
    deficiency, 8
Vitamin E, 116, 177

Xerophthalmia, 3, 6

Zinc, 11–12, 37–39, 187
    deficiency, 38–39
    role in development, 38